SEATED ACUPRESSURE THERAPY

From Ancient Art to Modern Practice
– a practical guide for therapists

SEATED ACUPRESSURE THERAPY

From Ancient Art to Modern Practice
– a practical guide for therapists

**Patricia Abercromby and
Davina Thomson**

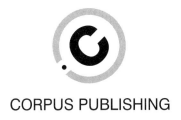

CORPUS PUBLISHING

Corpus Publishing Limited
PO Box 8 Lydney Gloucestershire GL15 6YD United Kingdom

Authors' note
As seated acupressure therapy has its roots in both China and Japan, we have recognized this by using both Chinese and Japanese symbols in the first two chapters.

Disclaimer
This publication is intended as an informational guide. The techniques described are a supplement, and not a substitute for professional tuition. Whilst the information herein is supplied in good faith, no responsibility is taken by either the publisher or the author for any damage, injury or loss, however caused, which may arise from the use of the information provided.

British Library Cataloguing in Publication Data
A CIP record for this book is available from the British Library
ISBN 1 903333 23 7

Acknowledgements

Davina Thomson: I am grateful to all my clients of seated acupressure therapy, who over the years have given me such satisfaction and made every day a new experience, often leaving me in awe with the profound and sometimes astounding results they have achieved from this therapy. I would also like to thank Patricia for her constant motivation and for always aiming for the summit.

Patricia Abercromby: We are both grateful to our families and friends who supported our efforts in putting this book together. I have benefited enormously from working with Davina whose experience in the classroom as a tutor, and as a working practitioner of seated acupressure therapy are arguably, unsurpassed in this branch of complementary therapy.

Additional Acknowledgements
Cash, Mel: *Sports and Remedial Massage Therapy*, Ebury Press.
Chaitow, Leon: *Muscle Energy Techniques for Muscle Dysfunction*, Churchill Livingstone.
Mercati, Maria: *Tui-Na*, Gaia Books Ltd.
Mochizuki, Shogo: *Anma*, Kotobuki Publications.
Schneider, Meir: *Self Healing*, Arkana Penguin Books.
Silk, Anne: *Air Quality and the Workplace of the Future*, Mid Careeer Press.
Williams, Tom: *Chinese Medicine*, Time Life Books.
Connelly, Diane: *Traditional Acupuncture, The Law of the Five Elements,* Traditional Acupuncture Institute.
Hix, S & Batten, J: *Fourteen Classical Meridian Charts*, Roswell Publications.

We are grateful to the above authors for aspects of their wisdom and works that have contributed to this book, and in addition, to Anne Silk and Polly Harper for their guidance, encouragement and contributions.

Photography Keith Spillett
Drawings Corpus Publishing
Printed and bound in Great Britain

Contents

Authors' Note

Seated Acupressure Therapy contains significant changes to our book that was originally published as *Seated Acupressure Massage* in 2001. We have modified the basic Kata to include some of the zero strain techniques pioneered by Gerry Pyves. The Archer's press has been replaced with the Scapula stretch, which we feel is much easier for the therapist to perform and there is no danger of tiring the wrist and shoulder joints, especially when working on several clients consecutively as we do at Exhibitions or in the corporate environment. We have also modified the arm stretch with a cradling stretch technique, which again takes the strain off the therapist's lower back and which the clients also seem to prefer.

We have also modified the leg acupressure routine to include work on the Liver, Spleen and Kidney meridians on the inside of the lower leg which we feel gives a more complete treatment as all the meridians on the legs are now stimulated.

Updated also are the statistics from the CBI and HSE on absenteeism caused by stress-related illnesses and we are pleased to include evidence from the first published clinical trial research on the benefits of Seated Acupressure treatments on a group of workers. (Rich, G. *Massage Therapy, The Evidence for Practice*, Mosby 2002)

Foreword

Some books are written to fulfil the author's dreams or ambitions whilst others are the result of a genuine need to tell the story or impart vital information. We believe that *Seated Acupressure Therapy* by Patricia Abercromby and Davina Thomson falls magnificently into both categories.

We have known Davina Thomson and Patricia Abercromby for several years and have visited their successful school on a number of occasions. They are both passionate about 'their therapy' and nothing is too much trouble to ensure they produce well trained and competent practitioners. This passion and eye for detail shines through this book, which is well produced and a fine balance exists between graphical detail and precise instruction. One can actually 'see' their students working as you progress through the easy to read pages.

Davina has been teaching various aspects of massage for many years and is an experienced teacher. For the last few years she has concentrated in running courses in Seated Acupressure Therapy ably assisted in both the administration and teaching by Patricia Abercromby, herself a qualified therapist and teacher.

The style of clothed and seated massage has gained popularity during the last ten years. The practitioner/therapist usually visits the workplace and many businesses find it beneficial for their employees, because it relaxes both mental and physical tensions thereby reducing stress and stress related problems and can create a measurable reduction in sick days.

This well written and illustrated book will be an excellent teaching aid to students and an aide-mémoire for the experienced practitioners. We found the chapters featuring the history of Acupressure Therapy and the basic understanding of Traditional Chinese Medicine very interesting and the section devoted to helping the therapist promote and market their newly acquired skills in the world of business completes the reader's education. Destined to be a best seller in this specialist market.

Shirley and John Beney
Founders of The Guild of Complementary Practitioners

Introduction

Seated acupressure therapy has entered into the culture not only as an acceptable modality in the corporate stress management environment, but also in the public sector. Go to any Health Fair or Exhibition and you will see seated acupressure practitioners working nonstop with a line of people waiting patiently for their 'turn.' In most major shopping malls, airports and fitness centres in many parts of the world, practitioners can be found demonstrating their skills on a willing and grateful public, and walk-in 'back rub' shops are opening up in many High Streets in cities and towns.

While it is a good development that so many people are willing to sit down on the ultra-comfortable therapy chairs and receive a treatment, it is vitally important that members of the public can be confident that their practitioner is fully qualified and insured to practice. In the UK, there are only a few training schools offering recognized and accredited training in Seated Acupressure Therapy that are fully accredited by the Guild of Complementary Practitioners. We would urge anyone who is considering training in this modality or any person seeking a treatment, to check the credentials of the training school and the qualifications of the practitioner offering the session.

We have included a detailed account of the routine that we teach in our school. There will be slight variations from sequences taught by other schools, but the basic Kata (a sequence of formalized moves) is instantly recognizable. Practitioners will find that working with clients sitting in the chair creates many possibilities for a variety of additional therapeutic and remedial techniques to enhance the basic sequence and to treat specific ailments, such as a range of overuse injuries. Some of our most frequently used additional techniques are included, but we are sure that you will have your own favourite and effective techniques to add to the list.

Marketing oneself as a practitioner is an area that, traditionally, challenges many of us. We have tried to give practitioners a few hints and tips on how to sell themselves and their services to a potentially vast client base. Also included are ways for practitioners to look after themselves and ensure that they stay fit and healthy. After all, we need to practice what we preach!

Although no book, DVD or video can ever be a substitute for attending a structured training course, we hope that the contents of the following pages will build on the knowledge of qualified practitioners of seated acupressure therapy and will inspire others to learn this exciting and dynamic skill.

Patricia Abercromby and Davina Thomson

Chapter 1
History of Acupressure Therapy

The seated acupressure therapy techniques that are taught and practised today have evolved from ancient East Asian massage techniques called ANMA in Japan, and ANMO in China. Anma translated literally, means press and rub, represented by the combination of Japanese characters for Anma.

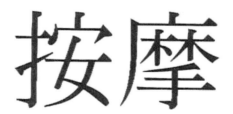

Japanese Anma script

This tradition has survived thousands of years of being passed down through generations building on their observations of Yin and Yang concepts, the Five Element Theory, (more of that later) meridians and acupressure points. Ancient writings from Japan indicate that Anma has its roots in India, Nepal, Tibet and Western China dating back 7000 years.

There is an interesting legend that the Chinese came to understand the power of acupressure points with the arrival around 10000 BC, of incredible seven feet tall healers known as the Sons of Reflected Lights. These beings could see the aura and the meridians of people with the acupressure points showing up as tiny pinpricks of light. They healed by directing their own life force at the sick person from a distance of several feet. Over the centuries, their sensitivity and power decreased and they moved closer and closer to the body until they were using the pressure of their fingertips, eventually graduating to acupuncture needles. Perhaps difficult to prove without any documented evidence but it makes a nice story.

Anma massage was first recorded in China during the Zhou and Qin Dynasties (1122AD – 207AD). During the Han Dynasty (221BC – 264BC) the legendary visionary, the Yellow Emperor Huang Ti referred to Anma and Acupuncture in the *Huang Ti Nei Ching* or the *Yellow Emperor's Classic of Internal Medicine*, now recognised as the oldest existing medical text in the world. Modern medical research has 'rediscovered' many of the medical observations made in this ancient tome and found them to be accurate. In the Huang Ti Nei Ching, it states that 'kidney supports bone', a truth somewhat lost on the Western medical establishment. This was until it was discovered that Vitamin D is an important factor in bone growth and more recently, that the chemistry of Vitamin D is changed in the kidney and provides the missing link in the control of bone growth and development.

Acupuncture became the treatment of choice for the Chinese nobility while the healers, or barefoot practitioners as they were known, travelled around from village to village offering Anma massage. Late in the Tang Dynasty which began in 618AD, the practice of Anma declined sharply but emerged later in Southern China as Tui-na, a form of Chinese massage that is growing in popularity in the West today.

In the early part of the fifth century, China started trading with Japan through Korea, and the Japanese were introduced to Buddhism and the art of Chinese medicine including Anma. In 718AD, a medical school was established in Japan to study acupuncture and Anma. More than 200 hundred years later, during which time many Chinese Buddhist monks and doctors emigrated to Japan, the oldest comprehensive medical text in Japan, the *I Shin Bo* was published in 984AD, covering all known medical subjects including Anma.

In spite of a decline in interest for a few hundred years between 1185 – 1574, the art of Anma survived and indeed flourished during the Monoyama period 1575 – 1602. Many new Anma techniques evolved during this time and were taught in the new medical schools that were established in Tokyo.

During the Edo period, 1602 – 1868 there was an exchange of medical knowledge with physicians who came to Japan with the Dutch Trading Company. The Dutch doctors introduced the Japanese practitioners to anatomy and physiology and in exchange, the Dutch doctors learned acupuncture and Anma and brought them back to Europe. Possibly as a result of this exposure to Western medicine, the powerful shoguns decreed in the middle of the 19th century, that only blind practitioners, who would have better developed touch sensitivity, should perform Anma for relaxation purposes. As the blind practitioners could not practise other forms of medicine such as herbalism, Anma massage came to be regarded as a poor person's health system and much technical and clinical knowledge was lost during this time.

Between 1868 – 1912, the shoguns fell from power to be replaced by an imperialistic government. Western medical practices became popular, to the detriment of traditional Oriental medicine. However, the blind Anma practitioners survived until the turn of the 20th century when the Japanese government of the day decreed that all Anma practitioners should be licensed and taxed. Many of them prudently reinvented themselves as Shiatsu (meaning finger pressure) practitioners to avoid the tax and licensing laws. In its early days a Shiatsu therapist performed only the Anma finger pressure but it has developed to include other areas of massage and Anma techniques. Shiatsu increased in popularity and was made more acceptable by Tamai Tempaku, a massage practitioner with a good knowledge of western anatomy and physiology and massage, who published a book in 1919 called Shiatsu Ho. In 1925, an Institute for Shiatsu was established by one of his students, Tokujiro Namikoshi. Massage was no longer restricted to the blind, and a more structured system of education and training was implemented for Anma and massage therapy. In 1964, Shiatsu was licensed as a therapy in its own right, independent from Anma.

Although Shiatsu evolved from Anma and both disciplines are similar in many respects, there are one or two differences to note. Anma utilises kneading and percussive movements not used in Shiatsu. Vibration techniques are used a lot in Anma but only occasionally in Shiatsu. Both techniques apply pressure to the acupressure points or tsubos, on the meridians.

Seated acupressure therapy is a hybrid of both modalities and was developed specifically for the workplace, hence the popular name of 'on-site massage' (a 15-minute massage routine developed by David Palmer, an American practitioner). In 1984 David was giving 15-minute massages through clothing to employees at Apple Computers in Silicon Valley in California. This was so well received that he went on to design a folding, portable massage chair. The chair has evolved into the light and portable model available today, providing total body support for the client and enabling the practitioner to give a more therapeutic and effective treatment.

In 1989, the sequence was being taught in the UK and since then it has continued to grow in popularity in many countries throughout the world. In its present form, the basic sequence or KATA (Japanese for dance), is recognizable in form, but varies from school to school, from a 15-minute massage routine to a 30-minute remedial and therapeutic treatment. It works on many acupressure points on the upper body, including shoulders, upper and lower back arms, hands neck and head. The basic sequence is instantly recognizable from the stance of the practitioner and from the meridians that are worked on. If a time machine could transport us back three thousand years to Japan or China, it is likely that the Anma practitioners of those times would recognize the modern seated acupressure therapy sequence on offer today.

Chapter 2

An Overview of Traditional Chinese Medicine

Seated acupressure therapy has its roots in ancient, traditional oriental massage techniques, and when practised with skill, accuracy and sensitivity, the sequence will help balance the flow of energy or Qi throughout the body, as the practitioner stimulates many acupressure points on the 12 major meridians. During training the practitioners will be introduced to the theories of Yin and Yang and the five elements, the conceptual basis of Traditional Chinese Medicine, of which acupressure therapy is an integral part. There are many excellent books available for those who wish to study this subject further. This chapter provides an introductory overview of the traditional Chinese view of health and disease, and hopefully, will give practitioners of seated acupressure therapy, a better understanding of the multiplicity of factors, physical, emotional and environmental affecting their individual client's state of health.

The major difference between Chinese medicine and Western medicine is that Western medicine is based on a philosophy that views disease either as a physical or mental problem. Although there is a general assumption that the two may be loosely connected, Western medical doctors, in tandem with the pharmaceutical industry, normally treat symptoms individually. Disease is approached from the view that it is caused by external factors such as invasion by bacteria or viruses or by degeneration of internal organs or systems of the body.

The philosophy of Chinese medicine is that everything in the Universe is part of an interdependent and mutually interactive energy force called Qi, where mind, body and spirit are merely different elements of the same life force and should not be considered separately.

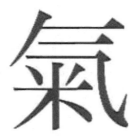

Universal Energy

Treatments seek to balance the energy dynamics, Yin and Yang, of the individual, by taking into consideration physical symptoms, emotional reactions and environmental factors. Thus a practitioner of Traditional Chinese Medicine (TCM), might use or suggest a combination of acupuncture, herbal remedies, Qigong exercises, meditation or a Feng Shui reading to bring balance and harmony to their patients' lives. The Chinese culture was one of the first to introduce preventative medicine where the wealthier patients visited their doctor when they were well, paying the doctor a retainer to keep them healthy. The doctor would lose his fee if his patient fell ill!

In spite of the radical differences between Chinese and Western medical systems, the two are not mutually exclusive, and elements of each can benefit the health of the individual. Practitioners of complementary therapies, including seated acupressure therapy, are uniquely placed to bridge the gap between the two approaches and can help broaden the philosophical and ideological basis of Western and Chinese medicine.

Yin and Yang

The concept of Yin and Yang is about balance between opposites. Universally Yin represents the feminine, quiet, substance and night while Yang represents the masculine, noise, function and day. In fact everything in

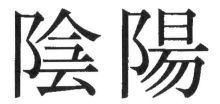 *Yin and Yang*

the universe, within or outside our bodies, even down to the food we eat, can be classified as Yin or Yang. In the body, disease is caused by an imbalance of Yin and Yang. Therefore, disease can be treated by correcting this imbalance and allowing the body to heal itself.

In the body there are 12 major meridians and 2 extraordinary vessels (the conception and governing vessels), each associated with an organ system or function. Meridians are paired in Yin and Yang, which is the representation of opposite but complementary qualities that are interdependent and are in a constant state of dynamic balance.

If one meridian has an excess of energy, the other will have a deficiency, so stimulating one or both can alleviate the imbalance. Qi circulates throughout all the meridians at certain periods during the day. For example, the lung meridian Yin, and large intestine Yang, are paired, or sister meridians. Blocked energy in either meridian can create an imbalance in the associated organ systems.

	YANG	**YIN**
In the world:	Sun Upper Hollow Positive	Moon Lower Solid Negative
In the body:	Spine/back Male Surface of the body	Chest/abdomen Female Interior of the body
In dis-ease:	Acute	Chronic

THE FIVE ELEMENT THEORY

The origins of Chinese philosophy, Taoism, developed through observation of nature and that everywhere in there is a deeper explanation of how Qi balances, interacts through the elements of Water, Wood, Fire, Earth and Metal, and supports all life forms. Within our bodies if this flow of energy is interrupted, disease can occur. From there, Taoists developed a medical system known as the Five Element Theory, the elements are the basis of all that exists. Each element is part of a larger cycle of Universal energy which is constantly moving.

Universal energy is regulated by the growth and control cycles. The growth cycle illustrates the way in which the elements and therefore the organ systems of the body support for one another; for example, water will promote the growth of wood and wood burns to create fire, etc. The control cycle counteracts the growth cycle and restores balance and harmony. Therefore, in the control cycle, water will control fire and fire in turn will control metal by melting it.

Five Element Theory Summarised

CREATION (Sheng) CYCLE

Fire creates Earth	The ashes of fire add to earth
Earth creates Metal	The expansion of earth creates metal
Metal creates Water	Metal separates, allowing water to flow
Water creates Wood	Water nourishes the growth of wood
Wood creates Fire	Wood builds fire

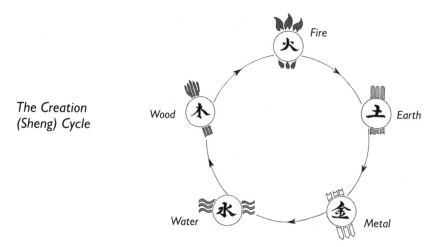

The Creation (Sheng) Cycle

CONTROLLING (Ke) CYCLE

Fire controls Metal	The heat of fire melts metal
Metal controls Wood	Metal can chop wood
Wood controls Earth	The roots of trees grow through earth
Earth controls Water	Earth can dam water
Water controls Fire	Water can dowse fire

The Controlling (Ke) Cycle

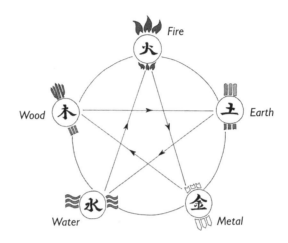

Element	**Paired or Sister Meridians**				
	YIN	(Abbreviation)	YANG	(Abr)	
Metal	Lung	L	Large Intestine	LI	
Water	Kidney	K	Bladder	BL	
Wood	Liver	L	Gall Bladder	GB	
Fire	Heart	H	Small Intestine	SI	
	Heart Protector/ Pericardium	PC	Triple Heater/ Triple Warmer	TW	
Earth	Spleen	SP	Stomach	ST	

MERIDIANS AND ACUPRESSURE POINTS OR TSUBOS

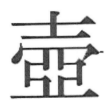

The meridians are a system of conduits that carry Qi or vital energy to every part of the body. The system involves twelve major meridians and two extraordinary vessels associated with an organ system with over 350 acupressure points and a further 250 non-meridian points (or tsubos). A tsubo, often translated as a 'jar' or 'vessel' is a point on the body where the meridian can be accessed more easily. Stimulating these points with finger or elbow pressure can remove the stagnant Qi that collects in the tsubos, thereby helping to balance the flow of energy throughout the body. Accurate location of the tsubos will obviously enhance the effectiveness of the treatment. Reference to the charts will help identify the locations of the points used in the treatment.

The 12 major meridians have the following number of tsubos or acupressure points:

Lung	11
Large Intestine	20
Stomach	45
Spleen	21
Heart	9
Small Intestine	19
Bladder	67
Kidney	27
Gall Bladder	44
Liver	14
Heart Protector	9
Triple Heater	23
Conception Vessel	24
Governing Vessel	28

There are eight extraordinary Vessels or pathways, connecting and collecting Qi which are not directly linked to organ systems but transfer energy to the major meridians as needed. The two most well known of these are the Governing Vessel and the Conception Vessel.

During a seated acupressure therapy session, especially if the legs are included, dozens of acupressure points on all the major meridians are stimulated to help balance the flow of energy throughout the body.

The meridians form two symmetric loops on either side of the body and energy flows through them in a well-defined, 24-hour circadian rhythm. Two further meridians are the Conception Vessel meridian up the front of the centre of the body and the Governing Vessel meridian, up the spine.

During the 24-hour cycle, there are specific times when there is a maximum flow of energy in each channel:

Lung Meridian	3 am – 5 am
Large Intestine	5 am – 7 am
Stomach Meridian	7 am – 9 am
Spleen Meridian	9 am – 11 am
Heart Meridian	11 am – 1 pm
Small Intestine Meridian	1 pm – 3 pm
Bladder Meridian	3 pm – 5 pm
Kidney Meridian	5 pm – 7 pm
Heart Protector Meridian	7 pm – 9 pm
Triple Heater Meridian	9 pm – 11 pm
Gall Bladder Meridian	11 pm – 1 am
Liver Meridian	1 am – 3 am

The received wisdom about emptying the bowels and not skipping breakfast makes more sense as it can be seen that the energy in the large intestine and stomach meridians is at its most active beween 5am and 9am.

FUNCTIONS OF THE ORGAN SYSTEMS

Lung

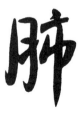

1. Regulates the secretion of sweat.
2 Regulates body hair and skin.
3. Respiratory conditions including asthma and coughing.
4. Eliminates noxious gases through exhalation.
5. Rules Qi and regulates Qi of entire body.

Large Intestine

1. Receives food and water from the small intestine and absorbs some of the fluids and excretes the remainder.
2. Removes stagnant Qi through excretion.
3. Supports lung in functions of respiration and immune system activities.
4. Storage and elimination of waste.

Kidney

1. Governs 'Jing' essence, the substance that underlies all organic life (a reservoir that nourishes the body and fuels the metabolism – jing is primarily inherited but enhanced by nutrition, exercise and lifestyle).
2. Governs bones and marrow and teeth.
3. Proper functioning of the ears.
4. Memory and concentration.
5. Harmonising sexual functions.
6. Survival and instinctual fear.
7. Regulate the amount of water in the body.
8. The gateway to the stomach.

Bladder

1. Transforms fluids through storage and excretion.
2. Helps to balance entire meridian system (through corresponding association points along meridian).
3. Addresses fear, depression, worry and agitation.
4. Similar charateristics to kidney.

Gall Bladder

1. Regulates the flow of Qi throughout body.
2. Governs decision-making process.
3. Influences the eyes, ligaments, tendons and joints.
4. Excess gall bladder Qi, may be shown as anger and deficiency as timidity and depression.

Liver

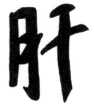

1. Maintains the harmonious movement of Qi throughout the body; known as the 'controller of strategic planning'.
2. The principal centre of metabolism – synthesising proteins, neutralising poisons, assisting in the regulation of blood sugar levels and secreting bile.
3. Harmonising emotions.

Heart

1. Governs the entire vascular system, controlling direction and strength of blood flow.
2. Nourishes tissues, removes toxins and influences all other organs.
3. Rules mental energy, known as Shen or Spirit.
4. Because of its importance it has a heart protector or pericardium.

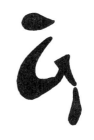

Heart Protector/Pericardium (Circulation Sex)

1. Protects the heart from external stresses – on a physical and emotional level.
2. Supports the heart in circulatory functions.
3. In charge of blood flow and sexual secretions.

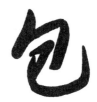

Triple Heater/Warmer

The triple heater is a function rather than an organ:

1. It transforms and transports Qi as it flows to all parts of the body and directs Qi to the organs, known as the 'Official of Balance and Harmony'.
2. Helps to transform and transport nourishment and to excrete waste.
3. Enhances the functions of the lymphatic system.

Small intestine

1. Responsible for receiving and transforming nourishment by absorbing food and drink.
2. Separating the pure or useful substances from waste products.
3. Assimilation of nutrients.
4. Rules discernment – involved in the sorting proces, the useable form unusable substances, both body and mind.

Spleen

1. Assists digestive process by transporting and transforming food.
2. Absorbing nourishment and sorting usable from unusable.
3. The primary organ in the production of prenatal Qi.
4. Ingested food and drink provide food Qi and creates postnatal Qi.
5. Governs blood, muscles, limbs and connective tissue – proper movement is dependent upon a well-balanced spleen meridian.

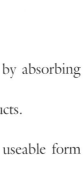

Stomach

1. Referred to as the 'sea of nourishment' in charge of digestion.
2. Transports food energy to all parts of body and nourishes muscles.
3. Whatever the disease, if stomach Qi is strong, the outlook is good.

The Governing Vessel is known as the 'sea of Yang channels', and influences all the Yang meridians and is used to enhance the body's Yang energy. It nourishes the brain and spine.

The Conception Vessel is known as the 'sea of Yin channels'. It influences all the Yin meridians and is important for the reproductive system, fertility, pregnancy and conception.

The two Extraordinary Vessels

They act as reservoirs of Qi for the twelve major meridians, filling and emptying as required.

Quick Reference Notes for the Twelve Major Meridians and Two Extraordinary Vessels

Conception Vessel (Ren) Acupressure Points CV 1-24

Yin – Starts midway between the anus and the genitals, runs in a straight line up the front of the body and ends at the midline below the lower lip.

Governing Vessel (Du) Acupressure Points GV 1-28

Yang – Starts midway between the coccyx and the anus and runs straight up the midline of the back, over the head and ends on the inside of the mouth at the junction of the gum and upper lip.

The Water Element

Bladder Meridian Acupressure Points BL 1-67

The Bladder meridian is the longest meridian in the body. Some of the bladder acupressure points on the back, **Shu** points, have direct energy links with other meridians or organ systems, all of which are stimulated during the seated acupressure massage sequence.

Yang – Starts on the inner corner of the eye and ends on the outer edge of the little toe.

Kidney Meridian Acupressure Points K 1-27

Yin – Starts on the sole of the foot and ends in the depression on the lower edge of the collar bone, two thumb widths from the midline.

The Wood Element

The Liver Meridian Acupressure Points LV1-14

Yin – Starts on the inner margin of the big toe at the base of the nail and ends between the 6th and 7th ribs, just below the nipple.

The Gall Bladder Meridian Acupressure Points GB1-44

Yang – Starts in the small depression at the outer corner of the eye and ends at the outer edge of the little toe at the base of the nail.

The Fire Element

The Heart Meridian Acupressure Points H 1-9

Yin – Starts in the centre of the armpit and ends on the base of the little finger on the inside edge.

The Small Intestine Meridian Acupressure Points SI 1-19

Yang – Starts at the outer edge of the little finger at the base of the nail and ends in front of the small piece of cartilage that forms the front part of the ear.

Heart Protector (Pericardium Meridian) Acupressure Points HP1-9

Yin – Starts on the chest on the lateral side of the nipple in the space between the 4th and 5th ribs and ends at the centre on the tip of the middle finger.

The Triple Heater (Sanjiao) Meridian Acupressure Points TH 1-23

Yang – Starts at the outside of the fourth finger at the base of the nail and ends on the outside tip of the eyebrow.

The Earth Element

The Spleen Meridian Acupressure Points SP1-21

Yin – Starts on the outer edge of the big toe at the base of the nail and ends 6 thumb widths below the armpit, between the 6th and 7th ribs.

The Stomach Meridian Acupressure Points ST 1-45

Yang – Starts just above lower edge of the eye socket in line with the pupil and ends on the outside edge of the second toe at the base of the nail.

The Metal Element

The Lung Acupressure Points LU 1-11

Yin – Starts in the space between the first and second rib near the shoulder and ends on the outside edge of the thumb at the base of the nail.

The Large Intestine Meridian Points LI 1-20

Yang – Starts on the outer edge of the index finger at the base of the nail and runs along the arm to the face ending at the outside edge of the nostril.

Chapter 3
Stress in the Workplace

Is the boss a Sabre-toothed Tiger?

Every era in the history of mankind has created different types of stress. Our early ancestors were mostly concerned with basic survival, finding food and shelter and fighting off predators. Facing a sabre-toothed tiger would certainly raise the stress profiles of the times, but at least the denizens of the caves could burn off the adrenalin and other stress hormones, either by running like the wind or by holding their ground and fighting for their lives.

Some stress is vital for our survival, otherwise we would not bother to get up in the morning. However, most people will agree that the advent of information technology and all the spin-offs from industry have pushed the vast majority of the working population into a state of constant high biochemical stress, with inadequate in-house strategies for reducing it. The result of some of these developments are measurable in the most recent surveys published. Statistics in the European Foundations Survey of working conditions in the European Union indicate that 30% of absences are due to back pain and 28% from stress-related conditions, resulting in 600 million working days lost per annum.

A quick trawl through the Internet revealed over 100,000 sites dealing with stress management in the workplace. The scientific and medical journals and the press have been devoting a lot of space publishing Government and privately funded research and surveys relating to RSI (upper limb disorders), computer vision syndrome (CVS) and other manifestations of stress-related illnesses. Clearly, a whole new industry in stress management is developing in response to the demand.

Stress Specifics

The stress word is bandied about quite freely these days. We talk about being 'stressed out,' and most people have daily experiences that are major causes of stress, such as a near-miss experience on the motorway on the way to work, or an agitated boss looking for sales figures. It is worthwhile reviewing the various causes and manifestations of stress both physiological and psychological, that clients may present with.

'Hard work never killed anyone' our grandparents used to say and that is probably true, however they were referring to physical work and not 8 hours in front of a VDU! It has been established that we all need a short break from any routine task every 90 minutes to stay healthy. In the office environment, sitting non-stop at a computer, possibly under flickering artificial light that throws glare and reflections onto the screen, and having lunch at the desk, is probably one of the quickest and most common routes to stress-related illness.

Legislation

Since 1989 there has been legislation in place introduced by the European Commission outlining basic provisions for Health and Safety at work, to ensure that employees are not harmed by the effects of work-related stress. The specific guidelines state that empoyers should:

- Aim to prevent work-related stress.
- Assess the risks of work-related stress by looking for pressures at work that could cause high or long lasting levels of stress and deciding who might be harmed.
- Take adequate action to prevent the harm.

While this is a useful guideline, it is important to remember that stress factors vary from person to person and that how we deal with the stress is more important than the situation itself. Therefore one individual may react differently to the same situation on any given day. This makes it extremely difficult for management to identify who may be harmed by pressures at work. Employers need to be aware of the two basic personality types:

1. Type A is prone to high levels of stress, being impatient, uptight and highly driven and frequently set high goals for themselves and others.
2. Type B is calm, reasonable and more laid back. Most people will have some qualities from both type A and B but recognition of which type predominates may help to assess their stress triggers.

Holmes – Rahe Stress Scale

This scale grades life's events and changes according to the amount of stress they cause. Arguably type A and type B personalities may react to a different degree to the same stress scale. If you have experienced changes giving you a total of over 50 in the last 6-12 months, then you may be experiencing some degree of stress:

1. Death of someone close   100
2. Divorce/separation   75
3. Separation   65
4. Injury/illness   53
5. Marriage   50
6. Redundancy/fired   47
7. Retirement   45
8. Pregnancy   40
9. Birth of a child   39
10. Change in finances   38
11. Argument with spouse   35
12. Child leaving home   29
13. Trouble with in-laws   29
14. Completing education   27
15. Trouble with boss   23
16. Change of work   20
17. Moving house   16
18. Going on holiday   15
19. Christmas   12
20. Breaking the law   11

Environmental factors too, contribute to stress levels, electromagnetic radiation from computer screens, artificial lighting, poor workplace ergonomics, noise, traffic pollution and overcrowding all take their toll. Needless to say, too many cups of tea and coffee, cigarettes, alcohol, recreational drugs, sugar and salt also create stress reactions, including increased output of stress hormones, nervous tension and fatigue.

What happens to the body during a stress reaction?

When faced with a challenge, the body responds biochemically in a way unchanged since the dawn of mankind. The reactions involve the brain, the nervous system and virtually every part of the body. There is an instant increase in the flow of adrenaline, cortisol and noradrenalin. Adrenaline speeds up the heart and respiration rate and increases muscle tension. Noradrenalin and cortisol create a feeling of excitement by raising blood sugar levels for quick thinking and for the extra energy needed to deal with conflict. Thyroxin stimulates the body to react quickly and endorphins act as natural painkillers. The digestive system contracts, the skin sweats and the mouth turns dry. These are all autonomic responses of the fight or flight mechanism and cannot be controlled voluntarily. This is great when the cause of the challenge is the tiger, or even when white water rafting. However, when this occurs in modern commercial life, the stress challenges may happen several times in one day. If there is no acceptable way to fight or run or to burn off the excessive secretion of hormones, people are left feeling tired, irritable, anxious, frustrated and susceptible to illness and infections. Medical research has shown that there are stress-related links to a number of serious and potentially serious conditions including:

- Cardiovascular ailments including high blood pressure, angina and coronary disease.
- Cancer.
- Strokes.
- Digestive problems such as irritable bowel syndrome, colitis and stomach ulcers.
- Asthma and allergies including eczema and psoriasis.
- Diabetes.
- Depression.
- Alcohol abuse.
- Computer Vision Syndrome (CVS) and other Repetitive Strain Injuries (RSI).

Apart from the personal misery caused by all of the above conditions, lost working days run into millions, and for a large corporate company, losing a single top executive to a stress-related illness can cost hundreds or thousands of pounds.

The more high-profile debilitating conditions such as repetitive strain injury and computer vision syndrome alone, are costing millions in litigation fees in the US, Canada and more recently in the UK.

Repetitive Strain Injuries (RSI)

What is commonly referred to as repetitive strain injury is not just a modern phenomenon or confined to keyboard users. Before the Industrial Revolution, 18th century scribes and notaries suffered from wrist tenosynovitis (inflammation of the tendons and surrounding sheaths, often caused by repeated strain or trauma). By the end of the 18th century, machines had taken over and the occurrence of RSI symptoms in workers was reduced. In the 19th century, the most frequently recorded sufferers were musicians and tennis players.

Today, RSI symptoms have been reported as affecting people across the board of modern working life. RSI can also be classified as carpal tunnel syndrome, tendonitis, tenosynovitis, bursitis, epicondyliltis, texters thumb and others! The main factors that can contribute to RSI are:

- Static and incorrect posture.
- Overuse.
- Working long hours.
- Previous injuries in muscles and tendons.
- Exposure to cold.
- Dissatisfaction with your job and stress.
- Poor ergonomics.

Workers who are particularly RSI prone include:

- Keyboard operators.
- Laptop users.
- Bank clerks.
- Switchboard operators.
- Supermarket cashiers.
- Waiters.

- Housepainters.
- Assembly line workers.
- Seamstresses.
- Hairdressers.
- Manual labourers.
- Children too, are beginning to show signs of the condition with the repeated use of the keyboard for computer games.

In the target-driven competitive environments of most modern workplaces, it is easy to see how people fall into the trap of over-riding the warning signs the body gives out, such as fatigue, tired eyes, aches and stiffness in joints and muscles. A classic example would be the keyboard worker sitting for hours in front of a computer screen with wrists flexed, elbows bent and shoulders hunched, using only minimal finger movements. This activity or lack of it, will cause tissue damage. One common painful condition is carpal tunnel syndrome, caused by compression of the median nerve, possibly at various points along its course from the brachial plexus to the fingers, and possibly lead to a painful condition referred to as Carpal Tunnel Syndrome (CTS). Anderseon et al 1994 define the condition as, '*a common painful disorder of the wrist and hand induced by compression on the median nerve between the inelastic carpal ligament and other structures within the carpal tunnel*'.

Practitioners can test to see if the client has CTS by applying Phalen's Test. The client places both elbows on the table with vertical forearms and wrists flexed. If the client experiences numbness and tingling within 60 seconds along the pathway of the median nerve to the thumb and fingers, the test is positive.

During the basic seated acupressure therapy sequence, the median nerve pathway is worked on, and this will help to relieve symptoms of CTS. However, the practitioner can spend longer working on this problem with the additional techniques that are taught specifically to relieve this condition. These techniques are described in a later chapter.

In 1988, to meet the public demand for information and help, the RSI Association, a registered charity with its head office in London, was set up to support people concerned about Carpal Tunnel Syndrome, and other RSI illnesses. Although the RSIA has since ceased to exist, their work

CARPAL TUNNEL SYNDROME

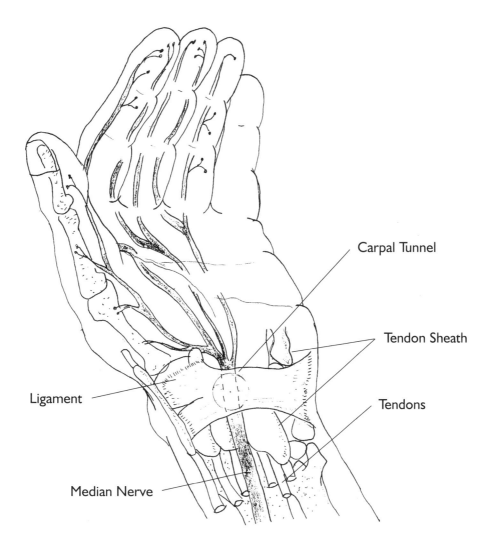

highlighted the distress that these painful conditions can cause workers and the practical advice and support that they offered sufferers set the standard for the current HSE legislation. Within that legislation is included the mission statement of the RSIA that employers should be working towards full recognition of the dangers of contracting RSI, minimising the risks to workers and seeing prevention as a priority. When the condition does occur in a worker, diagnosis must be accurate and effective treatment and rehabilitaion offered promptly, so that no one suffers long-term illness because of RSI.

Failure to observe this legislation can cost employers dearly. Since the 1990s there have been increasing numbers of claims going through the British Courts for damages. Around 240 major British companies have been sued by their employees for various work-related RSI injuries. Not all the claimants won their cases, but many did, and employers have been forced to pay out over £250,000 to some individuals. Proper workplace assessment, and regular breaks from the computer screen with some stretching and movement, incorporating a treatment programme, would in all probability, have saved companies litigation in some of the above cases.

- **Research in the US has shown that for every dollar invested in RSI prevention in an office environments, there is a return of $17.80.**
- **Organisations that employ strategies to improve work-place ergonomics have found that musculo-skeletal disorders (resulting in lost work time) were three times less likely to occur.**
- **Where employees thought that management showed understanding about balancing work and family responsibilities, encouraged skill development, involved them and treated them fairly, they were much more likely to be satisfied.**

Statistics from the TUC state that:
1 in 50 of all workers in the UK have reported an RSI condition, leading to 5.4 million working days lost in sick leave with six people in the UK leaving their jobs each day due to an RSI condition, bringing the cost to UK industry to around £20 billion annually.

There are many excellent books and information on the Internet offering guidance on the prevention of RSI (see recommended further reading).

Summary of Symptoms and RSI-Related Conditions

SYMPTOMS OF RSI
- PAIN – deep in the wrist radiating to forearm and shoulder – relieved by rest – worsened by resumption of repetitive activity
- Pins and needles of the hand
- Cramps
- Fatigue of arms
- Weakness, tendency to drop things
- Hands 'feel' swollen

WORK STATION ERGONOMICS

Screen distance approx arms length

15°

Screen eye level

Chair back supporting curves

90°

Sufficient Desk Space

Wrist rest (when required)

Feet flat on foot stool

Chairs to tilt pelvis forward

Adjustable chair height

- Disturbed sleep
- Irritability and mood changes

CLINICAL NAMES FOR RSI DISORDERS (work-related upper limb disorders)

Wrist and hand
- De Quervain's disease
- Carpal tunnel syndrome
- Trigger finger and thumb
- Guyon tunnel syndrome
- Ganglion

Forearm and elbow

- Epicondylitis (tennis and golfer's elbow)
- Tenosynovitis (flexorr or extensor)
- Pronator teses syndrome
- Radial tunnel syndrome
- Cubital tunnel syndrome
- Muscle compartment syndromes

Back and shoulders

- Rotator cuff or supraspinatus tendonitis
- Thoracic outlet syndrome
- Cervical spondylosis
- Bicipital tenosynovitis

Computer Vision Syndrome (CVS)

Another work-related injury that is receiving attention in the scientific journals and in the Courts, is Computer Vision Syndrome. Operators who use a computer screen for more than two hours every day, may experience symptoms now classified as Computer Vision Syndrome. Symptoms include:

- Eye irritations such as red, itchy or watery eyes.
- Tired eyes.
- Difficulty in focusing.
- Headaches.
- Backaches.
- Muscle spasms
- Contact lens discomfort
- Neck, back and shoulder pain due to poor posture.

Some 60 million people are suffering from eye problems due to computer work, with a million new cases being reported every year.

The human eye was not designed for staring at a computer screen. The image on the screen is made up of thousands of pixels or tiny dots and the eye is constantly trying to focus and make sense of these tiny images and the eye muscles for accommodation become tired. Also, with prolonged use and intense concentration on the project on the screen, people forget to blink as often, and the eyes dry out and become sore. Tests have proven that when working on a computer, individuals blink at less than half their normal rate. This in turn makes it more difficult to focus, causing blurred vision and possibly headaches and neck pain. To compound this problem, artificial lighting can cause glare and reflection on the screens. Not too many modern offices have adequate windows with far-reaching views of green fields and hills to give tired, sore eyes a much-needed visual break.

As with Carpal Tunnel Syndrome and other upper limb disorders, Computer Vision Syndrome can be avoided if sensible preventative action is taken. Practitioners should advise clients who use computers for more than two hours every day to practice the following good habits:

- Make sure the computer screen is 20 – 24 inches from your eyes at about 20 degrees below eye level.
- If you use a document holder, keep it close to the screen.
- Dim the overhead lights and keep desk lamps low and properly adjusted so the light does not enter your eyes or fall on the screen.
- Shifting. Every 15 minutes, focus on distant objects to relax your eye muscles.
- Palm your eyes. Rub your hands together to create heat. Lean your elbows on a table and gently cup your eyes without pressing your hands into your eyes. Close your eyes and breathe deeply and slowly, visualising that you are looking into blackness. This creates a profound relaxation of the internal and external muscles of the eyes (it quietens the mind too).
- Blink frequently to lubricate and sweep the eye clear of dust particles.
- Get into natural light as much as possible.
- When you sleep, ensure that the room is in total darkness to optimise the production of melatonin, a hormone which helps you sleep and keeps the biological clock in harmony.

This overview of 20th century stress, with the alarming impact that stress-related illnesses has, not only on industry but also on the health and well-being of millions of people in the workforce, underscores the valuable rôle that practitioners of seated acupressure therapy can play both in private practice and in the workplace.

Chapter 4

Why Seated Acupressure Therapy is the Ideal Therapy for the Modern Practitioner

There is no doubt that many employers are responding to the wake-up call from staff members demanding a better working environment. Human Resources departments are awash with new legislation designed to protect the employee from discrimination, unfair dismissal, and the right to sue if they sustain a work-related personal injury. Some large companies have on-site fitness centres, counselling services and Occupational Health Departments where nurses and a physiotherapist are on hand to treat sick and injured employees. The counsellors, nurses and physiotherapists all do a great job, but their work is reactive, as employees normally wait until a problem is debilitating before they make an appointment to be seen.

Fortunately, more and more enlightened employers are beginning to recognise the benefits of a direct 'hands-on' approach, and are allowing staff members to receive in-house treatment during working hours. Employees perceive this as a positive commitment of management for their wellbeing, and staff morale rises accordingly.

Almost any type of kindly touch has therapeutic value and the physical and psychological benefits of massage in particular are well documented. In 2002, a group of researchers conducted a clinical trial to investigate the physiological and psychological effect of on-site acupressure massage on a group of employees (*Massage Therapy, The Edvidence for Practice*, by Grant, J. Rich). During the eight-week study, two groups were used. The first was given a seated acupressure massage twice a week, the second control group took a break of 20 minutes to rest and lie down in a quiet room for the same periods. The results showed that the treatment group achieved the following results:

- Lower blood pressure
- Reduced anxiety and depression
- Increased feeling of emotional control and a positive effect
- Increased mental alertness
- Decreased sleep disturbances

What are the benefits of Seated Acupressure Therapy?

It is easy to see why seated acupressure therapy has become the treatment of choice for the workplace. It is quick, effective, clothes stay on, no messy oils are used, the massage chair is comfortable and supports the whole body, and afterwards the employee is relaxed, alert and ready to get back to work. People who would otherwise never consider having a massage because they are inhibited, too busy or just plain sceptical, are quite happy to have a treatment in the familiar surroundings of their own office building or gym. You can see the client's body visibly relaxing as the chair takes the strain off the spine and you encourage them to take a few deep breaths. (Shallow breathing is another symptom of stress).

Unlike the effleurage strokes of body massage, seated acupressure therapy works directly on the 12 major meridians and their associated organs and systems, balancing the flow of Qi or energy round the whole body. As a result, the tension in tight muscles and joints is eased, the circulation of the blood and lymph improves and the immune, endocrine and nervous systems all benefit. The rhythm of the 20 minutes of formalised moves, the Kata, promotes a sense of wellbeing in the client, leaving them calm and clearly focused, but more importantly, ready to tackle the rest of the working day with renewed enthusiasm! To summarise, the treatment will have the following effects:

- Relaxing and calming of the nervous system.
- A decrease in blood pressure and pulse.
- Relaxation of tight and sore muscles.
- Dispersal of toxins.
- Release of stagnant energy.
- Improved circulation of the lymphatic system, which strengthens the immune system.
- Improved alertness and concentration.

Consequently, there are many common conditions that will respond to and improve with seated acupressure therapy sessions. The list is long, but some of the most common stress-related ailments that practitioners encounter either in the workplace or in private practice include:

- Anxiety and depression.
- Backache and sciatic pain.
- Repetitive strain injuries such as carpal tunnel syndrome or frozen shoulder.
- Asthma and other breathing difficulties.
- Sinus problems.
- Eyestrain.
- Headaches/migraines.
- Insomnia.
- Chronic fatigue syndrome.
- Menstrual tension.
- Stress related muscle tension.
- Skin problems.
- High blood pressure * (see contraindications).

Screening the Client

As with any other complementary therapy, a full medical history should be taken before starting the treatment. Make sure that the screening is carried out in such a way that any potential problems are uncovered and discussed. Use your experience and powers of observation to help you ascertain if they are able to receive a treatment. Even if your client is booked in for a series of appointments, and you are familiar with their medical history, it is important to carry out a minimum screening to cover each session. Also at health exhibitions, charity events or corporate demonstrations when you may only have a short time with a client, the basic screening questions need to be asked and a disclaimer form signed by the client.

The following areas are either contraindicated or where special care must be taken, and the sequence modified accordingly: An asterisk appears beside questions that must be asked before any acupressure treatment *anywhere* is given, including short demonstrations.

Contraindications and 'Special Care' Conditions

- Women who are pregnant or trying to conceive should not receive any acupressure point work. Modify the massage work on the chair using some of the table massage effleurage – type strokes. It will still feel wonderful on the back, neck, arms, hands and head.**
- People with low blood pressure may suddenly feel light-headed and faint. *Be aware of working on people who are on medication to reduce high blood pressure, as this may lower it too much.* With permission and co-operation from the client's GP, it may be possible to have the client's BP monitored after treatments with the possible outcome of the medication being reduced if the blood pressure regulates naturally. If your client has low blood pressure, take the following precautions: *
- If the client has a history of fainting, or has low blood sugar or low blood pressure, make sure they have had something to eat earlier that day. If their blood pressure is anything more than slightly low, check with their GP. Check in with them during the treatment, and make sure that they sit up slowly.
- People recovering from recent surgery or who have been seriously ill must have consent from their doctor.*
- Do not work heavily on the lower back if the client has just had a large meal.
- Do not work on areas such as fractures, dislocations, and recent injections.
- Avoid treatment if the client has recently had alcohol or recreational drugs.
- Skin conditions such as psoriasis and eczema are not contraindicated if there is no broken skin – just avoid any friction moves. If the skin is broken, massage may still take place. However avoid the affected area. In infectious skin conditions, avoid contact.
- If the client has suffered an injury or trauma within twenty-four hours.
- Any communicable diseases such as influenza or tuberculosis.

Receive consent from their GP/specialist for the following conditions

- Epilepsy.
- Diabetes (they may have peripheral neuropathy).
- Cancer.
- Arthritis
- Any degenerative bone disease
- Thrombosis
- Hip or shoulder replacement surgery or metal plates in the body.
- If client is on medication

At the end of the screening process, ask the client if there is anything else they may want to ask before starting the session.

What to do if the Client faints or feels faint

Remain calm – get the client to lie down in the recovery position, or place their head between their legs. Give the client a glass of water. Do not leave the client whilst they are feeling unwell. Reassure them and ascertain a likely reason they may have fainted – i.e. an empty stomach, recent illness, low blood pressure, medication?

Preparation

If you have an appointment set with a client, make sure you arrive in plenty of time to set up your chair. Ensure that the room is a good temperature and preferably in a quiet, private area. Your body and mind also need to prepare to work on a client and a few minutes of stretching, Tai Chi or "Do-In" (awakening the body by working on the meridians with a loose fist) are ideal ways to prepare.

Loosen and stretch the arms, hands and fingers too before you start working. Too many massage therapists have to give up their profession early because they develop painful hand conditions that could be avoided with a good hand-maintenance programme. The following self-massage routine is based on the suggestions of Japanese Anma master and teacher, Shogo Mochizuki, and is ideal not only for massage practitioners but for anyone, such as keyboard operators, who have to make lengthy repetitive movements with the hands and arms.

1. Warm the muscles of the arms and shoulders with vigorous friction rubs and squeezes. Rotate the shoulders in both directions.
2. Place your arm on the table with your palm upwards. With the heel of your other hand on the medial border of the forearm, firmly squeeze and rotate the muscles of the forearm until they are warm and loose.
3. Percuss the length of the forearm with a loose fist or with the back of your other hand.
4. With your opposite thumb rotate the muscles of the wrist starting at the thenar side of the carpal bones (on the lung meridian). Apply the rotation by moving the whole hand, not just the thumb, and work your way round the wrist until you arrive back where you started.
5. Stroke firmly with the opposite thumb down the length of all spaces between the metacarpal bones from the wrist to the base of the fingers, back and front of the hand. Massage, squeeze and rotate the fingers of each hand with the thumb and index finger of the opposite hand.

Explaining the Treatment to a new Client

If it is the first time with a new client, an introduction and even a brief description of the therapy and some reassurance may be necessary. Some people may not have had any sort of massage before and may be slightly apprehensive. Don't be tempted to go into a long description about Yin and Yang and the Five Element Theory. If it is their first time, they are probably there more for the experience, so keep the explanation simple.

Show them how to sit in the chair, explain that they do not have to remove clothes and that no oils will be used. For their first treatment, most people are happy to hear that the treatment will make them feel better by relieving tension and stiffness in the back and neck and that they should feel more relaxed but energised and clear-headed.

During subsequent treatments, you can introduce more specific information about the effects of acupressure therapy if it seems appropriate for your client. Demonstrate how to sit in the chair and ensure the client will be comfortable – i.e. they have removed ties, belts, glasses, watches or items of jewellery if necessary and loosened collars. Treat personal effects respectfully and place them   nearby and make sure the client does not leave without them at the end of the session.

Screening

Ensure that you carry out the minimum screening, or take client notes. This is not only essential to ensure that the client is not contraindicated in any way, but complete notes will provide you with specific treatment details and feedback over a period of time.

Hygiene and Appearance

Ensure that you have a professional appearance, that your hands are clean, fingernails short and long hair tied back. It is not sensible or practical to wear white trousers or a white skirt or dress to give seated acupressure therapy. A white cotton top and dark, loose-fitting comfortable trousers always look smart and professional.

If you have badges from your training school and organization for complementary therapists, then wear them. You earned them through your hard work and it shows your client that you are a qualified professional. Some practitioners like to work in bare feet – this is acceptable in private practice but is not recommended in the workplace, wear sensible footwear.

Clean the chair and face rest after each client (in front of them) and wash your hands. Some practitioners like to use paper or towelling face covers on their chairs. If you choose not to use face covers, have a box of man-sized tissues handy in case your client is sensitive to the vinyl or leather, sweats a lot, or wears heavy make-up.

Music and aromatherapy burners may be appropriate, obviously depending on the venue, but be careful of your choice of oils, nothing too heady.

Client Comfort

Remain aware of body language – some clients may not want to tell you if they are experiencing discomfort. Check that the pressure is comfortable, especially when using elbow pressure on the back and thumb pressure around the occipital base. Ensure that they tell you at any time if they would like you to alter the pressure.

Practitioner Posture

Maintain a correct posture at all times, and use your body weight to apply pressure and stay relaxed – you will not tire yourself out as much and the pressure will be much more even. Maintain constant contact with the client and breathe from your Hara (centre just below your navel). Keep yourself grounded, letting the energy flow through your body and in turn, the movements will flow better.

Water for Practitioner and Client

Advise the client to drink a large glass of still water after the treatment. This is to flush any toxins that may have been released from the muscles into the blood stream and prevent stiffness (as they would if they had taken part in any sort of exercise). It is also very important that you, the practitioner, drink a glass of still water after each client to re-hydrate and to keep your energy levels up. Aim to drink a minimum of 2 litres of water each day for optimum health, more if you exercise.

Chapter 5

Seated Acupressure Therapy Sequence

This chapter gives a detailed step-by-step guide for practitioners who have trained or are undergoing training in seated acupressure therapy. We have included photographs for each move, and where necessary, we show the stance from a distance and a close-up of each move.

The following pictures illustrate the basic sequence or Kata. It is important to remember that although the work stimulates the flow of energy in the 12 major meridians, not all the points worked are tsubos or acupressure points. The Kata is a rhythmical sequence of moves designed to balance the flow of energy to all parts of the body and throughout the session, many tsubos *are* directly stimulated with thumb and elbow pressure.

The Chair

Most chairs come with a carry case. This not only makes the chair totally portable, but ensures that the chair stays looking good for longer, particularly if your work entails client visits, keeps the chair clean and is more hygienic.

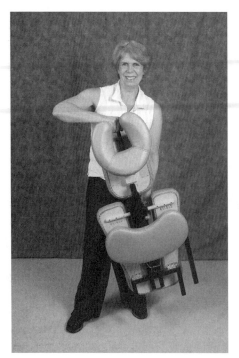

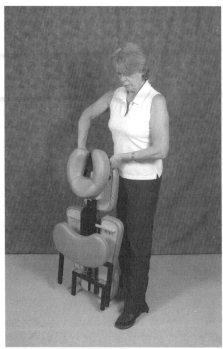

Remove the chair from the case and stand it upright.

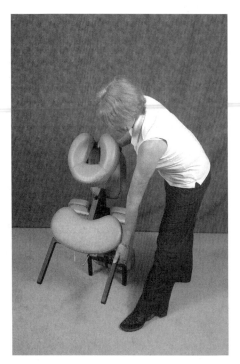

Move the 'A' frame out on the chair.

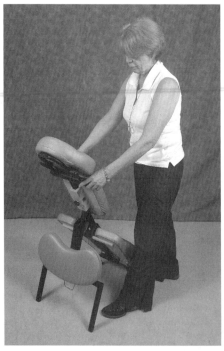

Pressing the knobs simultaneously on either side of the cross-bar, just above the chest piece, will allow you to raise the head rest.

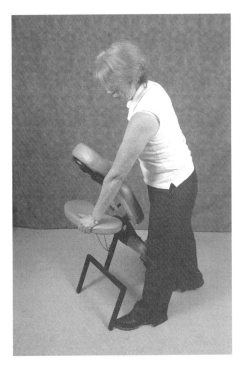

There are three positions for the armrest. Select the position most suitable for you and your client.

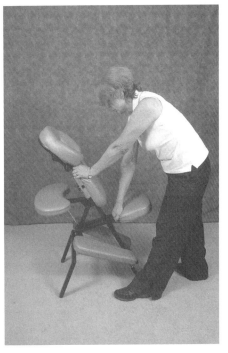

Raise the seat to the correct height for you and your client and ensure that it is secure.

Centre

Before you start work on any client, take some time to centre yourself. This allows you to become more focused and grounded. Once the client is in the chair, place your hands on their shoulders ask them to take a deep breath and drop their shoulders.

Brush down the back twice, then run your thumbs down either side of the spine lightly and slowly, taking the opportunity to check for any curvature and muscle tension.

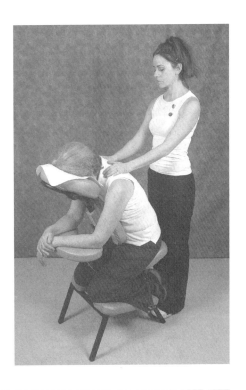

Double Palm Press: *(five positions, twice)*

Place one foot behind the chair, front knee slightly bent and the other straight on the ball of the foot ready to shuffle back between each pressure. Place your hands on either side of the spine, arms straight, thumbs pointing upwards. Start as high up on the thoracic spine area as your height will allow.

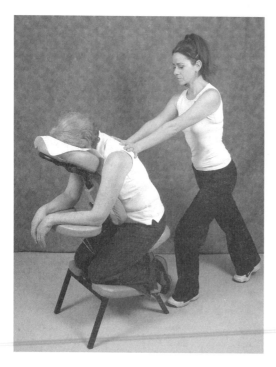

Ask your client to "take a deep breath and continue breathing deeply and evenly". Flex your front knee and allow your body weight to transfer itself through your arms to the client's back as they breathe out. The pressure should be at 90 degrees to the client, with downward pressure for the last position.

This is the first firm contact with the client, it gets them used to your touch, opens the back for further work and encourages deep breathing.

Double palm press

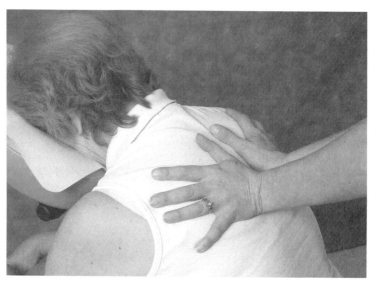

It is important to keep both arms straight as this helps the energy to flow freely and enables the practitioner to let their body weight sink through their arms. Remember to shuffle back with the back foot as you move down the back, this helps to keep your back straight as you work. For the last pressure, you may reinforce this, using both hands as shown.

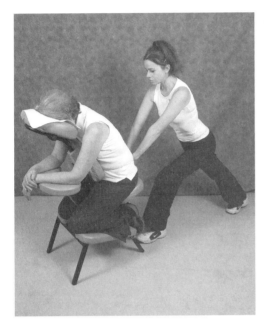

*Move down
the back*

Reinforced hand press

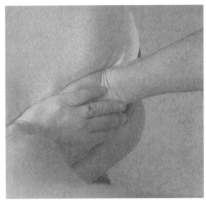

Scapula Stretch: *(three positions, twice)*

Stepping round with your left foot to the left side, place the left foot in front and keep the right leg back straight in line with the spine. Looking straight ahead, shoulders facing forwards, flex your left knee moving the muscle away from the spine with your forearm.

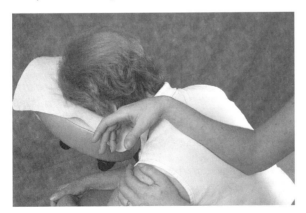

Scapula stretch

Forearm Press: *(three positions, twice)*

Keeping your left hand on the shoulder, place the underside of your right forearm at the junction of neck and shoulder. Let your body weight sink into three points across the top of the trapezius, starting as close to the neck/shoulder junction as possible and ending just in front of the acromion process, remaining on the muscle. This move should be slow in both applying the pressure and releasing.

You may need to move your own legs slightly closer together, as it is easier to get above the client and sink down into the top of the trapezius, rather than trying to use your strength. Ensure that you angle your arm slightly, turning your palm away from you to use the fleshy part of your forearm.

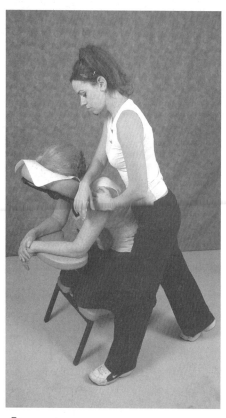 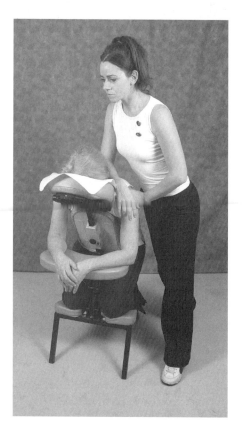

Forearm press

Erector Spinae: *(nine points, twice) Small Intestine SI 14 and Bladder Meridians BL 11-18*

Place your right leg in line behind the client's spine, stand on the ball of the right foot. Position the elbow in point 1, located about one inch away from the spine between C7 and T1; this is SI 14. Relax the wrist keeping the elbow at right angles to the client's back. As the elbow bends, allow the pressure to sink gradually into the point, by bending your front knee. Come in half an inch closer to the spine for points 2 to 9, which lie in the spaces between the vertebrae. Shuffle your back foot back between points.

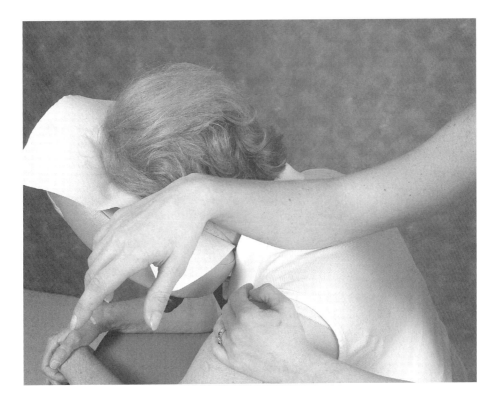

Always go more gently on the first line of points to assess the pressure. It is important at this point to check that the client is comfortable with the pressure. It is quite a common mistake for practitioners to stay too far away from the spine, this will lead to discomfort as the pressure is then applied to the head of the ribs. Make sure you are close to the spine along the erector spinae muscles, but not actually on the spine.

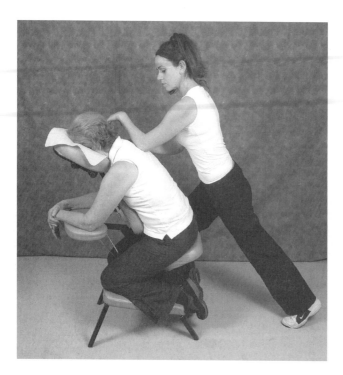

Make sure that you lift the pressure off as you shuffle back with your back leg, move down the erector spinae muscle, one vertebrae at a time to point 9. Points 2-9 are on the bladder meridian

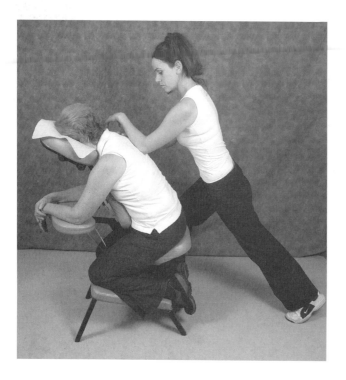

Scapula Medial Border: (Elbow Work) *(four points, twice) Small Intestine SI 13 and Bladder Meridian Bl. 39, 39, 41*

These points are on the medial border of the scapula starting roughly level with T1 and moving downwards in a straight line, ending in line with the inferior angle of the scapula. Point 1 is SI 13. Move in closer to the spine for points 2,3 and 4 on the bladder meridian.

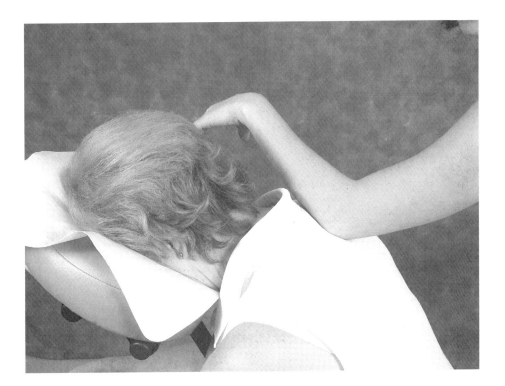

Trapezius Crest: *(three positions, twice) Gall Bladder Meridian GB 21 and Large Intestine Meridian LI 16*

Make sure you start very close into the neck and try to get above the points to allow your weight to sink in. Point 2 is GB 21. Point 3, LI 16 is in the depression behind the acromio-clavicular joint.

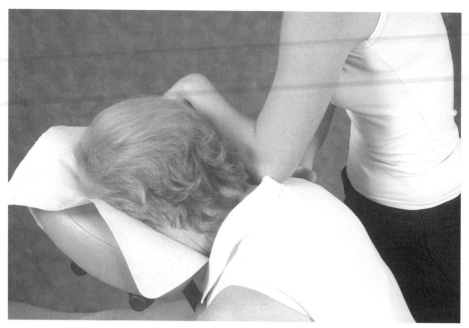

Place your elbow on the trapezius crest close to the neck. Allow the elbow to sink into the first point, moving outwards.

Scapula to Sacrum Rub and Brush Down

Using the heel of the right hand, rub in a vigorous circular motion on the erector spinae muscles, from the shoulder to sacrum. Brush down.

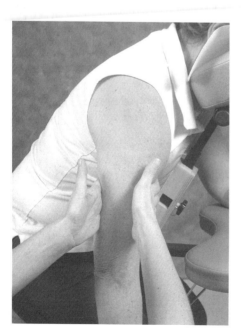

Posterior Upper Left Arm

Kneel or squat as you lower the client's arm giving it a gentle downward pull.

Hold the top of the arm with both hands and rub down to the wrist twice.

Arm Squeeze

Squeeze the whole length of the arm in five positions, starting at the deltoid muscle and ending at the wrist.

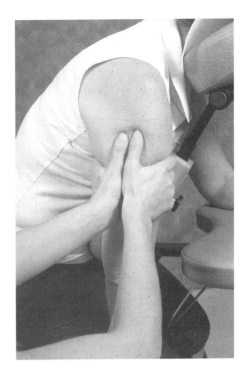

Deltoid to Elbow *(five points, twice)*

Point 1 Triple Heater Meridian
Point 5 Large Intestine Meridian

To locate the first point, let your thumb slide off the head of the humerous and down into the deltoid in the slight depression at the top of the arm. With your thumbs, using a hand over hand technique 'Walk' down 5 points to the fifth point just above the elbow crease on the lateral border of the triceps muscle, ending above the elbow in line with the client's middle finger.

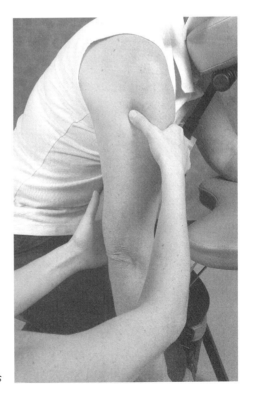

First of 5 Points

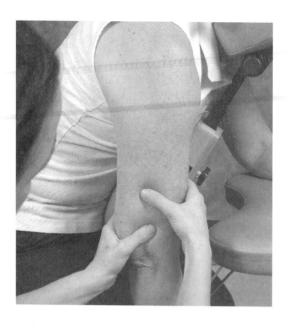

Hand over hand technique to Point 5

POSTERIOR LOWER LEFT ARM

Radial line *(five points, twice)*

Large Intestine Meridian LI 11, 9, 7, 5
(five points, twice)

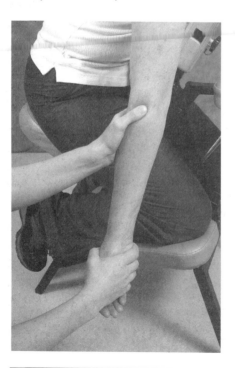

Turn the hand so that the thumb is facing you. Locate Point 1 on the radius just below the elbow crease in the brachioradialis muscle. This point, L.I. 11 can often be tender, particularly if the client has tennis elbow or RSI type symptoms.

LI 11 is often tender

Point 5, LI.5 is located midway between the tendons of the extensor pollicus brevis and longus muscles in the crease of the wrist. If you are working on the left arm, use your right thumb to apply pressure.

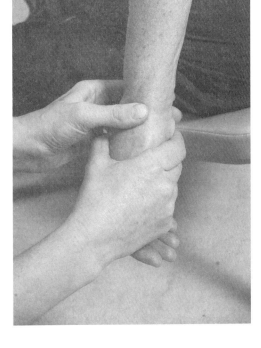

Point 5

Triple Heater Meridian: Points 9, 5, 4 (also known as Triple Warmer or Sanjiao Channel *(five points, twice)*

Turn the hand so the back of the hand is facing you. Starting just below the elbow, apply pressure to five points between the radius and ulna, end on the wrist.

Point 5 TH 4 lies in the depression between the tendons of the extensor muscles in the transverse crease of the wrist. In the middle of the wrist joint

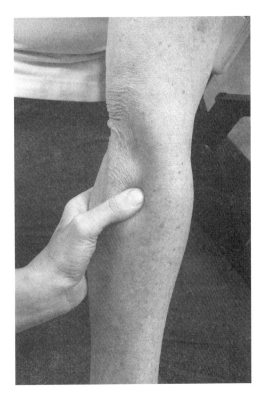

Triple Heater Meridian

Ulna line *(five points, twice)*

Small Intestine Meridian: Points SI 8, 7, 6, 5

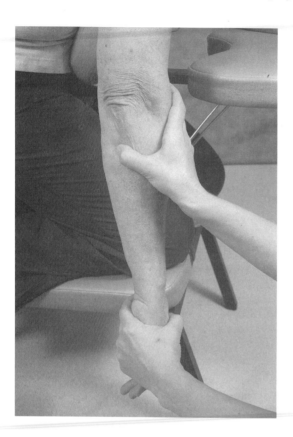

Turn the hand so the little finger is facing you and press SI 8 (below the elbow in the groove under the medial epicondyle), and work down in five positions, finishing at the end of the ulna bone at the side of the wrist. This point, SI 5 lies in the depression between the styloid process and psiform bone.

1st of 5 points

HANDS

Wrist Squeeze

Squeeze the sides of the wrist twice, with your thumb and forefinger as you walk around to the front. Place the arm back on the rest.

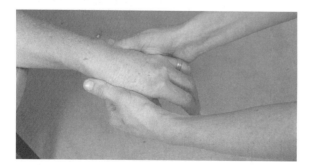

Hand Spread

Using the heels of your hands, firmly spread the back of the client's hand.

Thumb Strokes and Mobilization

With your fingers supporting the underside of the client's hand, use your thumbs to stroke down twice firmly between the outer metacarpals, turning your thumbs towards you and finishing between the fingers.

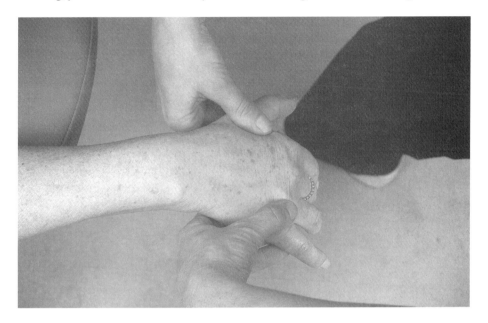

Follow with two mobilizations, once again ending through the fingers. Repeat thumb strokes and mobilizations down the inner metacarpals.

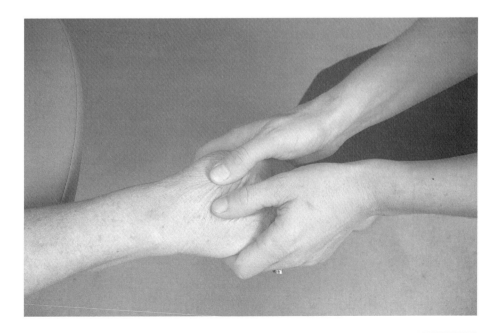

Great Eliminator (LI 4)

Squeeze twice between the client's thumb and index finger for a few seconds, gradually easing into the point and increasing the pressure if appropriate. This can sometimes be very sensitive as it is a powerful elimination point, which can help with headaches, constipation and detoxification.

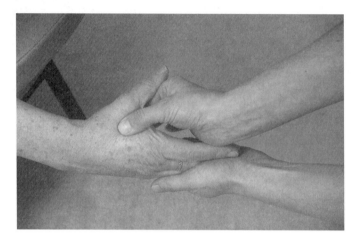

Great Eliminator, Large Intestine 4

ANTERIOR LEFT ARM AND INNER HAND

Heart Meridian H. 3, 4, 7 *(five points, twice)*

Turn the arm over, and with your right thumb press five points starting below the elbow on the inside of the arm (H3) and ending on the wrist. Points 4 and 5 are H4 and H7.

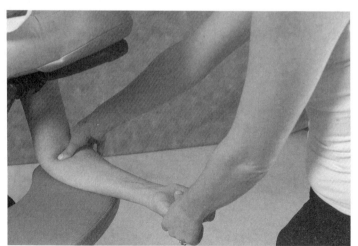

Heart 3

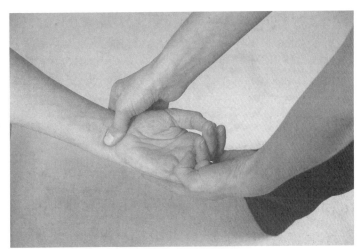

Heart 7

Heart Protector Meridian HP 3, 4, 6, 7 *(five points, twice)*

Point 1 is located just below the elbow crease in the middle of the anterior forearm.

Apply thumb pressures down five points starting in the middle of the arm just below the elbow and finishing in the middle of the wrist. Keep your arm straight while you work and use your body weight to lean into the point.

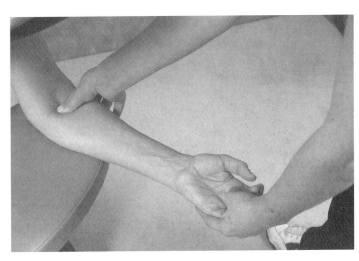

Heart Protector Meridian

Lung Meridian *(five points, twice)*

Starting on the outside crease of the arm below the elbow, press five points ending at the wrist.

Stroke Down

Stroke down twice from elbow crease to the fingertips to open and relax the hand.

Palm Spread

Using the heels of your hands and thumbs, firmly spread the palm of the hand. This feels great, particularly if the client operates machinery or uses the keyboard for much of the time.

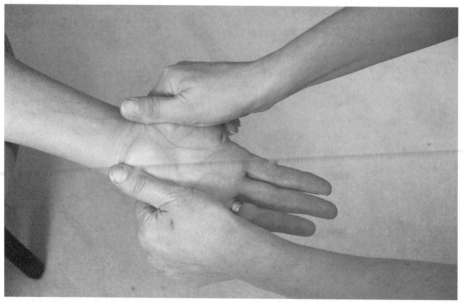

Palm Spread

Thumb Strokes and Mobilization

Stroke twice firmly down the palm of the hand between the outer metacarpals, finishing between the fingers and repeat. Follow with two firm mobilisations, once again ending through the fingers. Repeat thumb strokes and mobilizations down the inner metacarpals.

Lung 10

Apply pressure with your thumb in the middle of the first metacarpal bone to the centre of the thenar eminence, located on the fleshy pad on the palm side of the thumb.

Lung 10

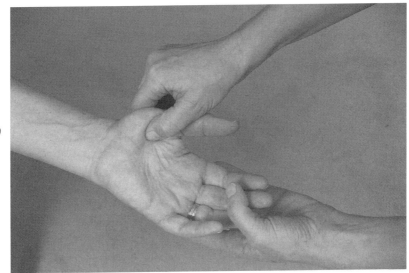

Coin Rubs

Using your thumb and forefinger, rub top and bottom of the thumb from base to tip and then rub down the sides.

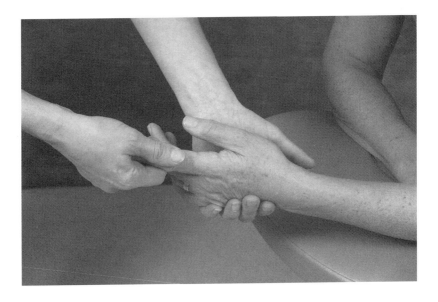

Squeeze the edges of the nail. Adopt a comfortable stance and make sure your back is straight.

Six meridians end or start at the fingers. Yin meridians: Lung, Heart Protector and Heart end on the fingers, Yang meridians: Large Intestine, Triple Heater and Small Intestine start on the fingers.

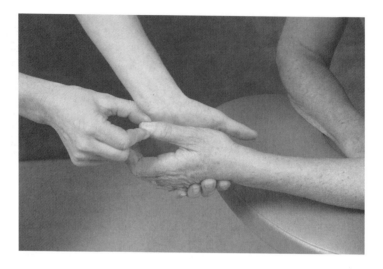

Finger Flicks

Sandwich the tip of the finger between the first phalangeal joints of the index and middle finger. Press the tip of the thumb against the index finger to stabilise and pull off. You should hear a satisfying 'click'. The direction of the 'Flick' should be away from your own body. Repeat for each of the fingers.

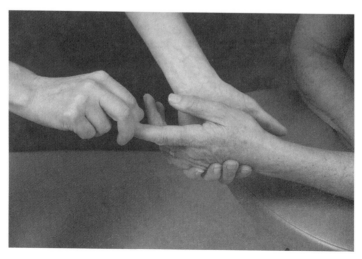

Arm Stretch

Gently but firmly cradle the client's arm and ask the client to take a deep breath and on the out breath, raise client's arm up and slightly away from their body, this will stretch the infraspinatus, teres minor and supraspinatus muscles. Hold the stretch for a few seconds and gently vibrate the arm.

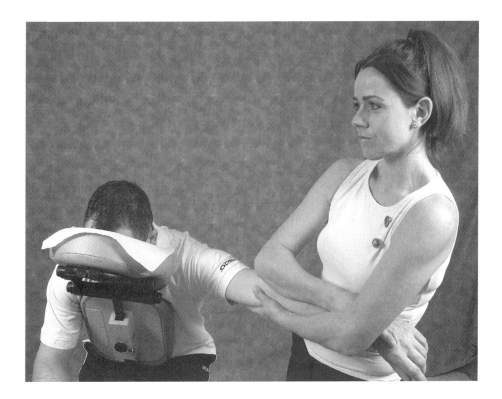

Gently lower arm and squeeze the left shoulder with your left hand as you walk round in preparation for the Scapula stretch.

RIGHT UPPER BACK AND SHOULDER

Repeat all the moves from the left arm to the arm stretch on the right side, reversing the hands used.

Lower Back

For the initial pressures on the lower back, if you wish you can repeat the move for the double palm press as carried out at the beginning of the sequence, however concentrating on the lower back area with a downward intention for points 4 and 5. This is recommended for clients with very sensitive lower backs, or use this method for the first of the two lines.

Alternatively, for a more focused pressure:

Loose Fist Pressure *(five positions, twice)*

Brush down twice. Keeping your arms straight, front leg flexed at the knee and back leg straight, stay on the ball of the foot. Your hands should be in loose fists, either side of the spine, starting around the mid to low thoracic area.

Ask the client to breathe deeply and on the out-breath drop the weight in through your arms by bending your front knee. The pressure should be on the flat area of the fingers between the knuckles and the first phalangeal

Loose fist pressure

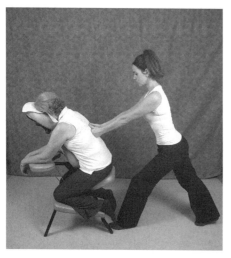
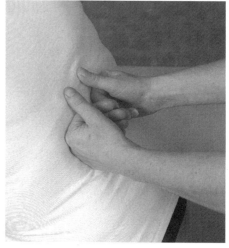

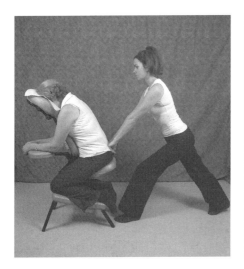
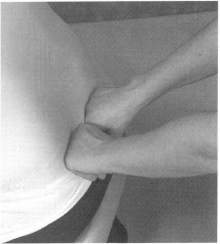

joint. Shuffle back with your back leg as you move down the spine. Work in five positions down the length of the lower back, and for the last pressure below the sacrum, turn your fingers to point downwards, stretching the back down to relax the lumbar spine.

Bladder Meridian BL 19-28 and BL 48, 29, 34, 35

Place your thumbs on either side of the spine, with the first point located in the erector spinae muscle, just between thoracic vertebrae 9 and 10. Move down between each vertebrae for 9 points.

Flex your front knee and apply pressure into the point steadily and evenly. Work down to L5 in the inter-vertebral spaces. You may also use your knuckles and for experienced therapists, your elbows, one side at a time.

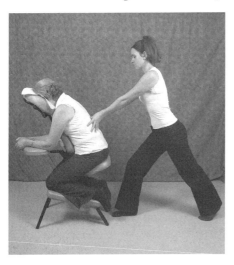
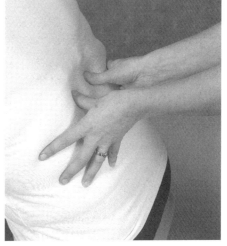

The last point should end between Lumbar 5 and Sacrum1.

As you move down the lower back with thumb pressures, your stance will widen. Always keep the back leg straight.

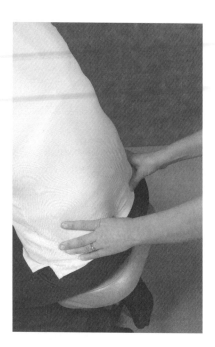

The first sacrum point is located at the sides of the sacrum on the soft tissue. Follow the shape of the sacrum in for points 2, 3, and 4 keeping on the muscle. The 4th point, Bl 35 is located above the coccyx on either side of the sacral vertebrae. This can help release lower back tension.

Gluteal Release

Squat or kneel behind the client. Using the heels of your hands with fingers pointing upwards, work in small circles from the sacrum outwards along the gluteus medius to the pelvic blade. Repeat the circles further down from the gluteus maximus to the hip joint. You may also use loose fists and for remedial treatments, work in deeper using the elbow.

Stand up and brush down from shoulders to sacrum.

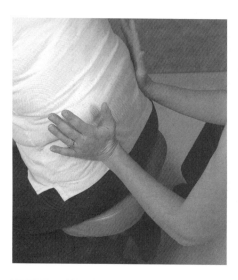
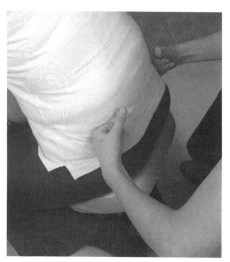

NECK

Base of Skull

Place your left hand on the top of the client's head and ask them to look down to stretch the neck. Press up into the underside of the occipital base starting just left of centre, in five positions ending behind the mastoid process. Check the pressure and work gently on the last point as this can be very tender.

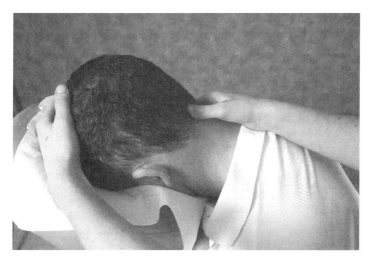

1st Point left of Centre

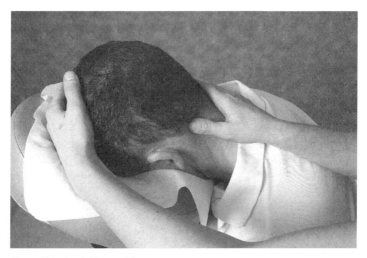

Point 5 behind Mastoid bone

Neck Lines *(three lines, five times each, twice) Governing Vessel GV 15 and Gall Bladder GB 20, 12*

Starting close to the cervical spine between C2 & C3, use the pad of the thumb to move the muscle away from the spine and keep your thumb pointing towards you. Gently rest your fingers on the other side of the neck and be careful not dig the thumb in. Continue down for 5 points to C6 and C7, repeating each line twice. Move further away from the spine by approximately one thumb width, depending on the width of the neck, for the start of each new line.

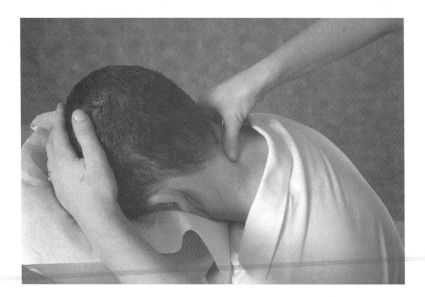

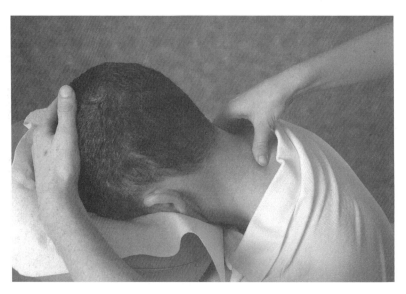

Trapezius Crest Points Small Intestine SI 15

Stand facing the back of the client and starting laterally, move in along the trapezius crest for 3 points.

These three points are found on the crest of the trapezius moving in towards C7. The middle point is half way between the spine of the scapula and C7. Two of these points are trigger points and will often be tense and in spasm. Working on these points can help release tension in the trapezius muscles and also helps move blocked energy.

Squeeze the left shoulder as you move round the back of the client to the right side.

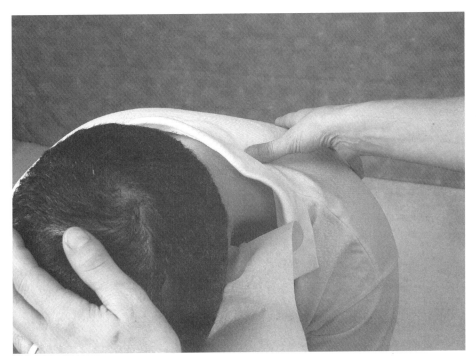

Work lateral to medial

Repeat all neck moves on the right side

Squeeze the right shoulder as you move to the back of the client.

Brush down twice.

Ask the client to take a breath and slowly sit up with their arms by their sides.

Gently hold the client's head above the ears to centre them. Give a gentle upward lift.

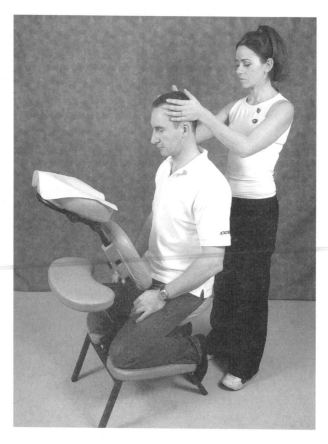

Neck Stretch

Stand directly behind the client with your feet hip width apart. Stretch the left side of the neck first, by placing your left forearm, palm facing upwards on the clients' left shoulder. Bring your right arm around so your fingers are placed on either side of the left ear.

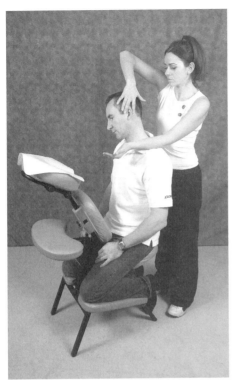
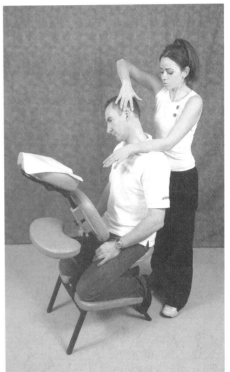

Ask the client to take a deep breath, and as they exhale, pronate your left forearm and press down on the trapezius. With your right arm, gently stretch upwards. You should be using about 70 percent downward pressure and 30 percent upwards.

It is important not to let your elbow rest on the client's head as you are stretching the neck. Hold the stretch for at least 5 seconds and release slowly. Repeat on the other side.

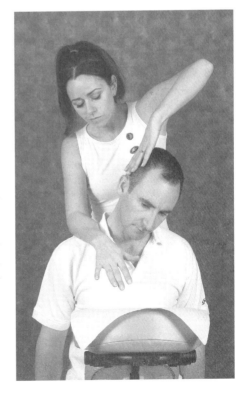

Scalp Massage

With the pads of your fingers and thumbs, massage in small circles moving the scalp. Make sure you stay away from the temples as this can be painful.

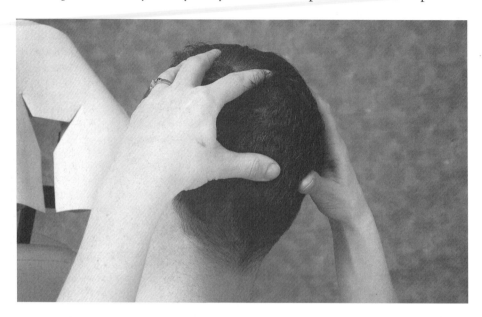

Scalp Lifts

With the pads of your fingers and thumbs, firmly and briskly, lift your hands off the scalp to stimulate the flow of blood to the head.

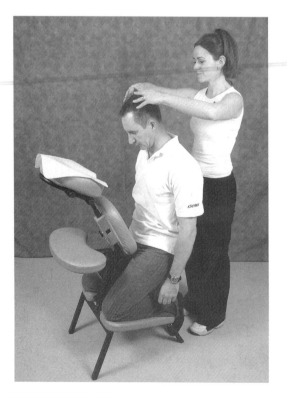

Cupped Hand Percussion

Clasp your hands together keeping a pocket of air between them as this creates a cushion effect for the client. If you have not perfected this yet, then work very gently!

With your wrists and hands loose, start from the occipital base, just left of the centre line and move up to the front of the hairline at the forehead and around the crown. Work all around the crown in a full circle to the front again. Finish by working downwards, just right of the centerline, bringing your hands off together at the occipital base. This move stimulates the gall bladder meridian.

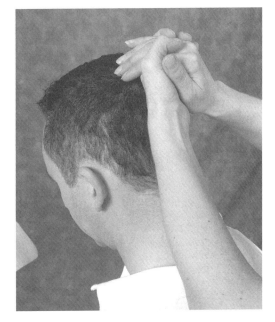

Double Forearm Press

Start with your forearms, palm facing upwards, resting on the trapezius close to the neck. Stand with your feet facing outwards and ask the client to take a deep breath.

As they exhale, drop your weight down by flexing your knees and apply pressure for 3 seconds and then in two further positions along the trapezius as you pronate your forearms for one second each as you rotate and repeat.

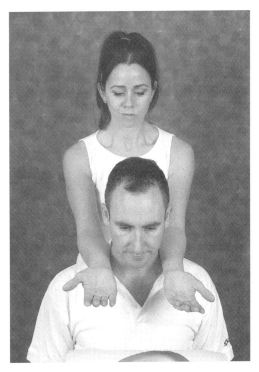

Palms facing upwards.

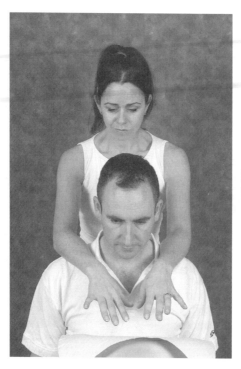

Pronate your forearms.

Thumb Squeeze Rotation

Starting on either side of the 1st thoracic vertebrae, squeeze and rotate thumbs in a circular motion and petrissage outward along the trapezius.

Then work down on either side of the thoracic vertebrae with your fingers still gently resting on the top of the shoulders.

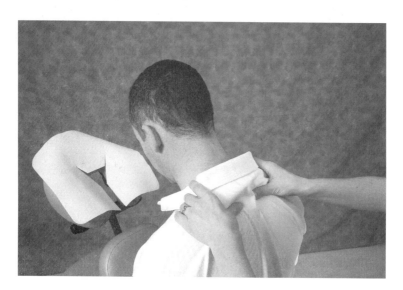

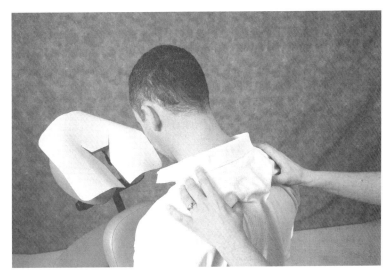

*Rest fingers
on shoulders*

Shoulder Squeeze

Squeeze the top of the trapezius in three positions, moving outwards towards the deltoid. Lift the muscle as you do this, taking care not to pinch.

Repeat.

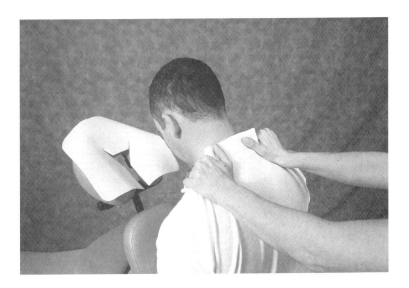

Then squeeze down the upper arm along the deltoid, lifting the muscle away from the bone.

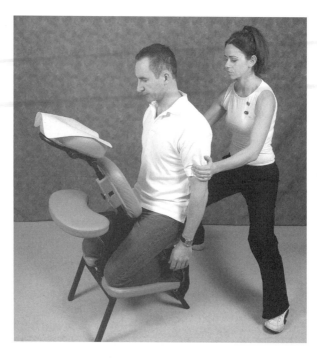

Squeeze down the upper arms.

Chicken Wing Stretch

Slide your hands down the client's arm and take the back of their forearm so the palms of their hands are facing forwards.

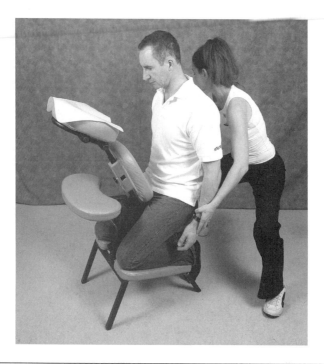

Ask the client to take a deep breath, and as they exhale, drop their head forward. As the client breathes out, raise their arms behind them, keeping their elbows pointing out at 45 degrees. Ask them to tell you when they can feel a good stretch and hold for 8 seconds.

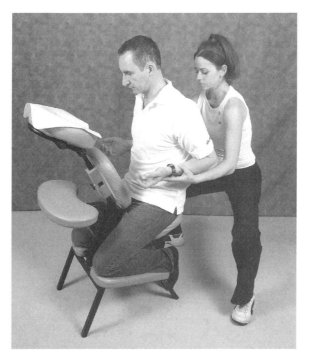

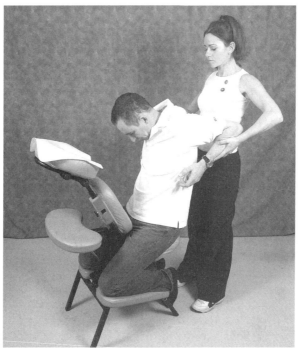

Hold stretch for 8 seconds.

Full and Final Brush Down

Place your hands gently on the client's head and let the energy gather for a moment.

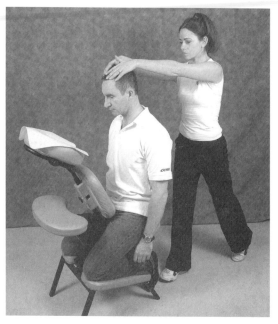

Sweep briskly down the back, repeat two more times and then once down the arms.

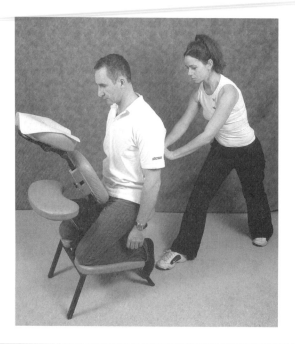

Shoulder Lifts

Take the arms at the deltoid, taking care not to pinch. Say to the client "Take a deep breath and when I drop your shoulders, let your breath go".

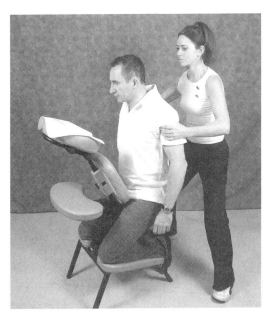

Lift the client's shoulders and gently 'throw' down their arms. Repeat this. On the third time, lift their arms, but just let them drop ready to go straight into the percussion.

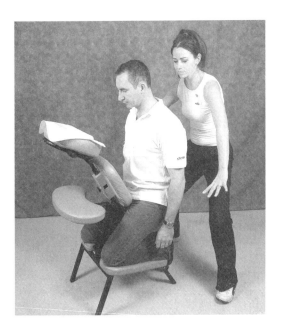

PERCUSSION

The following percussion moves should only be carried out over soft tissue and not directly on the bone.

Loose Hacking

As the client's shoulders drop, begin the percussion either side of the spine and work across the shoulders. Keep the wrists loose and the fingers apart, hack down to the mid-back. Bend your knees, keeping your back straight. Percussion will stimulate the circulation and help energise the client. Work along the trapezius and down either side of the spine, back up and repeat.

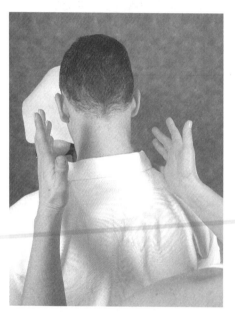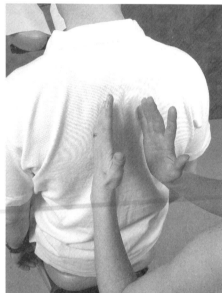

Hacking

Praying Hands

Start on the left shoulder, close to the spine, sandwich your hands together keeping your fingers apart and loose. Raise your elbows outwards to 90 degrees. Make sure you do not work directly on the spine. Move along the trapezius and down the left hand side of the spine. 'Jump' over the spine and up the right side and over to the right shoulder. Move back down the right side jumping the spine again and continue up the left side and back along the trapezius. Repeat.

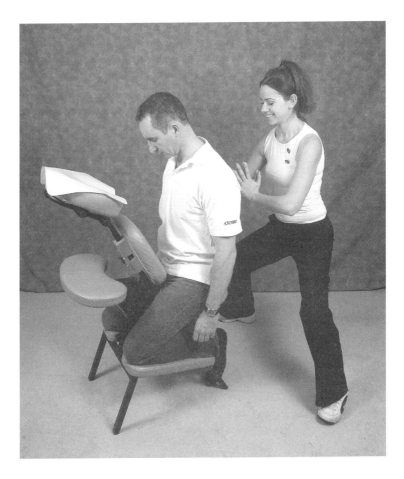

Praying Hands

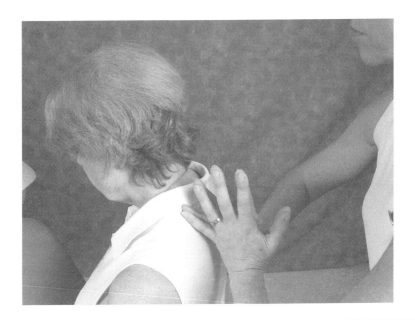

Cupped Hands

Place one hand over the other as if you are holding a small ball. Try to keep your hands airtight as this will offer a cushioning effect to the client. As with all the percussion moves, keep your wrists loose and follow the same route as before.

End the cupped hands with stitching, i.e. zigzagging from one side of the back to the other which integrates both sides of the back.

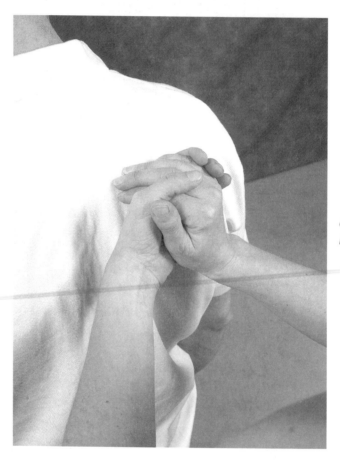

Cupped Hands

Place your elbow at the base of the spine and cup your hand gently over the spine, making a "channel" with your third finger and heel of your hand, so there is no direct pressure on the spine.

Using your elbow as a lever, keep your wrist soft and cup your hand a few times over the solar plexus area of the back. This stimulates the lungs.

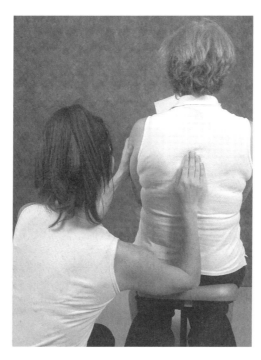

Cup your hand over the solar plexus area.

Grounding

Run your hands down the arms to the hands, and press the inside of the middle of the palm on Heart Protector or Pericardium 8

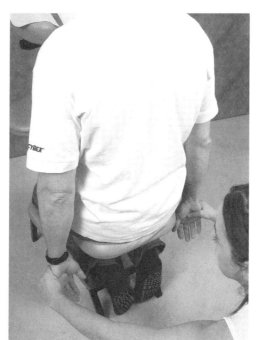

Heart Protector 8.

Apply pressure on the inside of the Achilles tendon on the kidney point to ground the client. Your thumbs should be facing each other on the kidney meridian.

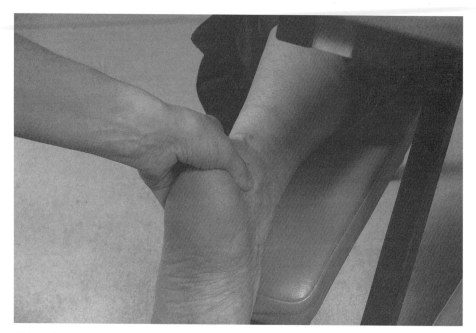

Kidney 4.

Walk round to the front and wait for them to open their eyes.

THE MERIDIANS

Anterior Arm Meridians (Heart, Heart Protector/ Pericardium and Lung Meridians)

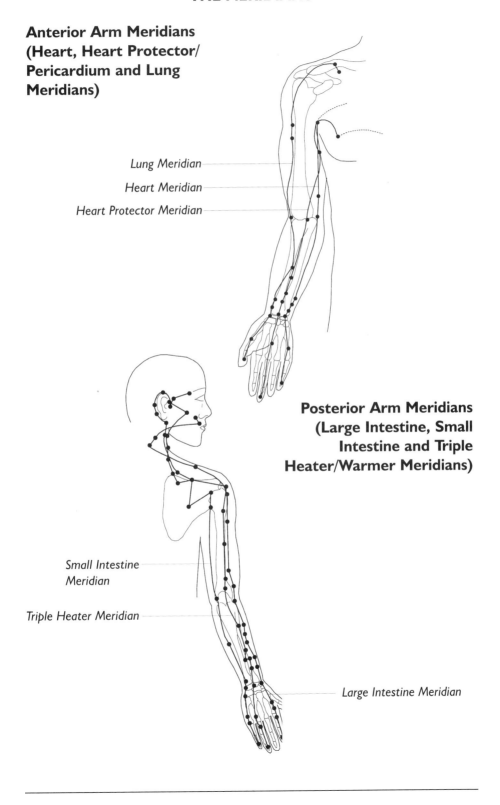

Lung Meridian

Heart Meridian

Heart Protector Meridian

Posterior Arm Meridians (Large Intestine, Small Intestine and Triple Heater/Warmer Meridians)

Small Intestine Meridian

Triple Heater Meridian

Large Intestine Meridian

Stomach Meridian

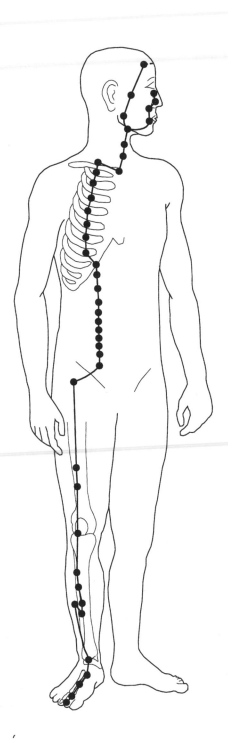

Bladder Meridian

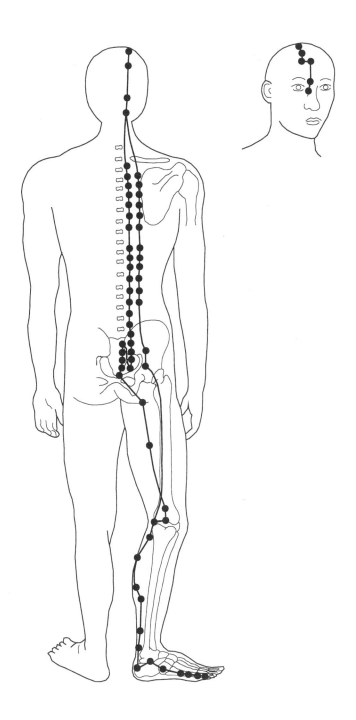

Gall Bladder Meridian

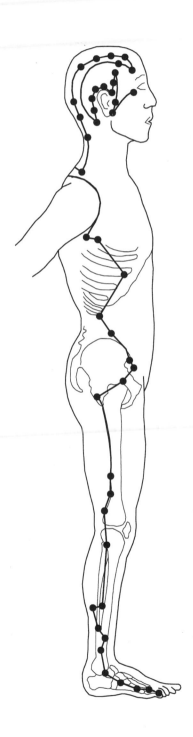

Kidney, Liver and Spleen Meridians

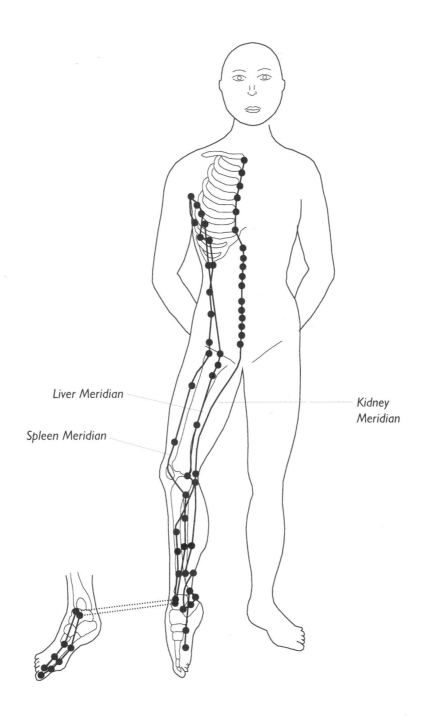

Liver Meridian

Spleen Meridian

Kidney Meridian

The Twelve Major Meridians and Two Extraordinary Vessels

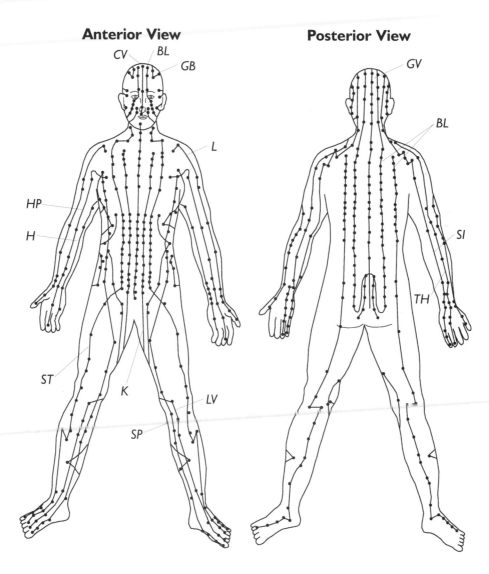

Anterior View

Posterior View

KEY

BL	Bladder
GB	Gall Bladder
L	Lung
LV	Liver
SP	Spleen
K	Kidney
ST	Stomach

H	Heart
HP	Heart Protector/Pericardium
CV	Conception Vessel
GV	Governing Vessel
BL	Bladder (inner and outer line)
SI	Small Intestine
TH	Triple Heater

Chapter 6
Additional Techniques and Stretching Exercises

LEGS

Although the chair lends itself to treating the upper body, we have found that the legs can very easily be included in a regular treatment and still keep the flow of the session. The best time to include the leg sequence is just after the lower back work and before the neck. It can be equally important to include the legs for the following reasons:

- There are additional meridians on the legs, which are not included anywhere else in the treatment.
- A sedentary lifestyle can lead to poor circulation and lack of movement in the lower body.
- Lower limb injuries can be prevented and treated by freeing the energy pathways and large muscle groups in the legs.
- Lower back problems including pelvic tilts and can be alleviated by working on the legs.
- Pre and post event sporting activities can benefit from this work.

The main focus is to maintain the rhythm and timing of the treatment when working on the legs by keeping the flow of the rest of the sequence. As you will see from the diagrams, there are 6 major meridians that flow through the legs:

- Stomach
- Gall bladder
- Liver
- Spleen
- Bladder
- Kidney

The main focus is to first warm the meridian pathways, using either the heel of the hand or forearm (on the stomach and gall bladder); and by squeezing and warming the other meridians – first on the upper leg and then the lower leg. Once the areas have been warmed, then if you wish, and time permitting, work into the points with either your elbow, thumb or finger pressure.

To maintain the rhythm of the sequence, we work in 5 positions on both the upper and lower meridians:

1. Warm stomach meridian; 5 positions using heel of hand or forearm. Start gently as this can be a very sensitive area.

   Gradually increase the pressure as the area becomes less tender – repeat as many times as necessary. If the client has lower back problems, this may be noticeably more sensitive on one side than the other.

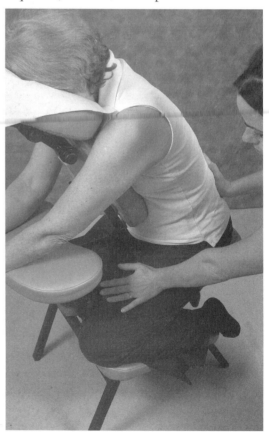

2. Warm gall bladder meridian; 5 positions using heel of hand or forearm. Repeat as required.

3. Work into 5 points on stomach meridian using elbow or thumb pressure.

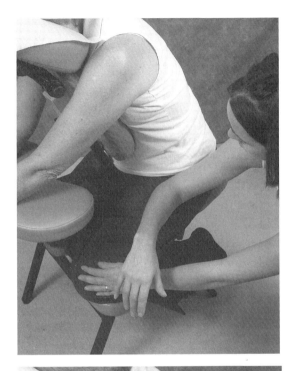

Use elbow or thumb pressure.

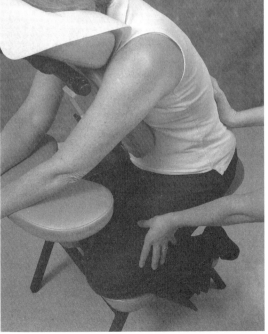

4. Work into 5 points on gall bladder channel using elbow or thumb pressure.

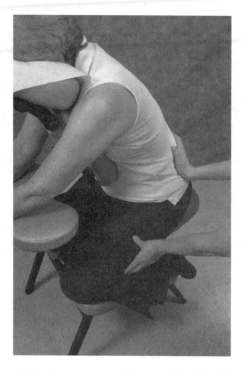

5. Lower the leg off the chair and rub and warm the muscles from knee to ankle, taking care to work on the inner leg as well as the back of the leg.

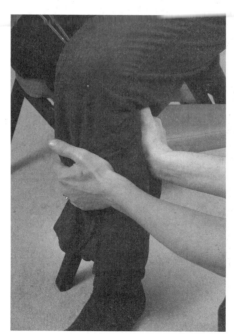

Warm muscles.

6. Start with the stomach meridian, and work 5 points using you thumb. Work from just below the tibial tuberocity (lateral and inferior to the patella) in five equidistant points to just in front of the lateral maleolus (ankle).

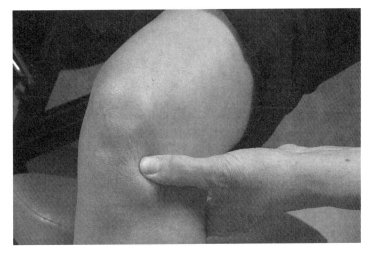

Stomach Meridian.

7. 5 points on the gall bladder meridian from below the knee along the peroneal muscles to the calcaneofibular ligament, just below the ankle bone.

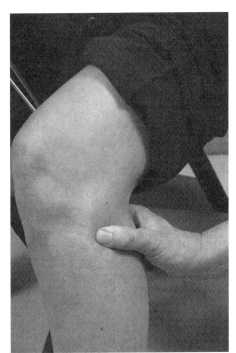

Gall Bladder Meridian.

8. 5 points down the bladder meridian using either your thumb, index or middle finger from behind the knee to the Achilles tendon.

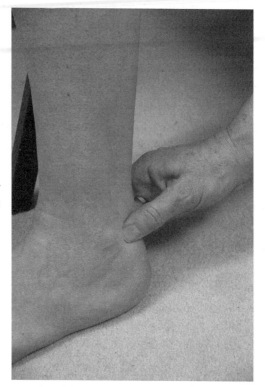

Bladder Meridian

9. 5 points down each of the 3 meridians on the inner lower leg, starting from the anterior (liver and spleen) and working to the posterior (kidney). There is some cross-over on the liver and spleen meridians – however pressing these points will ensure that many of the tsubos or acupressure points are stimulated whilst still retaining the flow of the sequence.

10. Brush down leg and squeeze the foot before replacing on rest.

ARMS AND HANDS

You will have read in our earlier chapter on 'Stress in the Workplace', how debilitating repetitive strain injuries and upper limb disorders can be. Of course prevention is better than cure; however, if a client develops RSI type symptoms, we have included some of our tried and tested treatment methods. Just by carrying out the acupressure therapy sequence, you will be addressing many of the areas that RSI can come from – neck, shoulders, arms, hands and wrists. Here also are some more specific remedial techniques that will allow you to concentrate on these areas. We would recommend that you increase the treatment time accordingly, allowing time to include some of these techniques in addition to the usual sequence on the neck, upper back, shoulders, arms and hands.

Dragon's Mouth Technique

Make each hand into the shape of a "C" with your fingers and thumb. Keep your hand firm and work down the triceps, biceps, and deltoid, easing the muscle and soft tissue away from the bone. Move rhythmically down the upper arm, gradually increasing the pressure as the area become easier. You may notice congestion (a dimpling effect), and the area may go red – this will increase the circulation along the median nerve route to the elbow. We are not focusing on the problem area – on the contrary, we are working around the area of pain, to improve circulation to the affected tissues. The client may notice the arm becoming warm and also experience a tingling sensation. If the client already has RSI symptoms, they may feel a certain level of discomfort. We always work within the comfort zone of the client – it is better to see the client twice a week for 2 weeks, than try to over – treat the area in the first session.

Points worked during this will include Triple Heater 10, just above the elbow joint on the posterior upper arm, which is useful in treating arm and elbow pain, Small Intestine 8, 9 and 10, on the triceps, for treating frozen shoulder, elbow and neck pain and Large Intestine 15, on the deltoid muscle, LI 11 just below the elbow joint on the medial side and LI 10 which is point 2 of the five points on the Large Intestine meridian on the posterior lower arm.

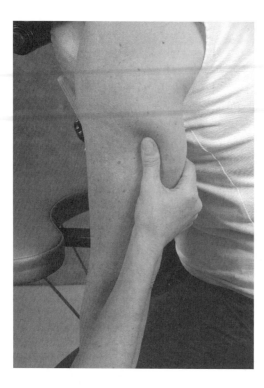

Dragon's Mouth Technique

Arm Nerve Stretch

This is a good stretch for anyone with symptoms of carpal tunnel syndrome or any other upper limb repetitive strain disorder.

With the arm by the side of the client, turn their hand, so that their thumb is pointing to the back of the chair, until you can feel a resistance. Keeping their hand under gentle tension, (get feedback) straighten their fingers and pull down to stretch. Hold for 15 seconds.

Alternatively, support the arm above the elbow and perform the same technique.

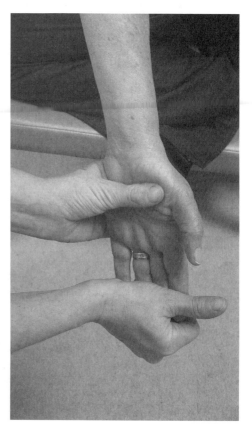

Wrist Release

Hold the arm just above the wrist with one hand and with the other, interlock your fingers with the client's and rotate the wrist firmly, but slowly and gently in both directions using slight traction. Gradually increase the size of the circle and work in both directions. Give a pull and shake.

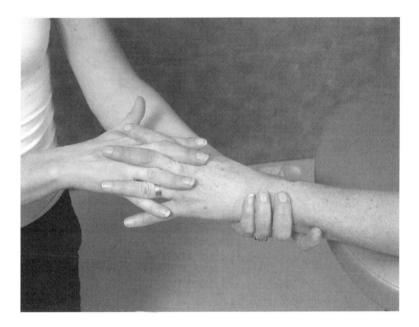

Wrist Release

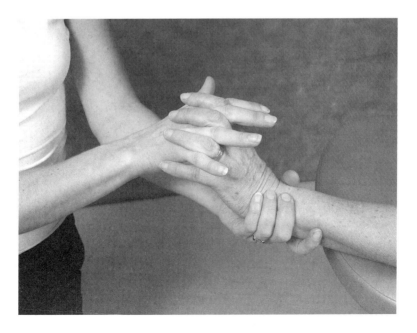

Caterpillar Walk

Using your thumb, walk along the tendon up the triple heater meridian. Use a variety of tissue releasing techniques, including friction and skin rolling on Triple Heater 5, which is above the dorsal wrist crease, in the depression between the radius and ulna bones. This can often be tight, and releasing this point helps frozen shoulder, carpal tunnel and RSI. (It is the 4th point that we work on this meridian during the arm sequence).

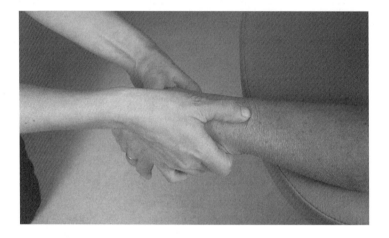

Palm Stretch

Using both hands, interlace your fingers with the client's fingers (whilst their hand is palm up), spreading the palm open. Work on points with thumbs. The stretch is more effective if you cross both of your little fingers over the client's middle finger.

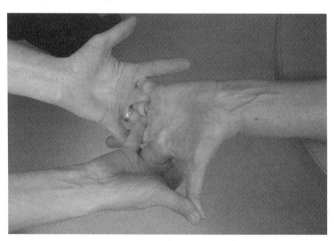

Palm Stretch

ADDITIONAL TECHNIQUES TO INTEGRATE WITH THE SEQUENCE

Sometimes you may wish to vary the treatment and integrate it with some different techniques and focus on specific problems.

The following techniques can all be carried out with the client sitting in the chair. While the basic treatment is profoundly effective as a stand-alone therapy, practitioners who have skills in other modalities will discover that they can integrate aspects of other therapeutic treatments into the session. We have given you a few of our favorite extra techniques that will add considerable therapeutic value to your sessions. Common sense and experience will guide you as to where they can be included in the sequence but we have indicated where to integrate some of them.

Whole Body Analysis

If you are giving a longer session and the client has specific problems, take note of areas of tension - and take time to make a quick assessment of the client, which will form a basis for attention to any problem areas.

Observe alignment of whole body. Is one shoulder or ear higher than the other? Is one side of the pelvis higher than the other or rotated forward? Check how the client stands. Is one foot further forward? Is the head turned more to the left or right than facing straight ahead? Are there any curvatures on the spine? Are there areas of hypertonicty on the back muscles? Use this initial evaluation to record details on your client consultation form. This will give you your own report from which you can refer back to and notice and record any changes over a course of treatments.

Warm Up

Single Palm Press

Use this technique at any time during the sequence to loosen tight back muscles.

Move to the left side of the client, and with the heel of your right hand, fingers pointing outwards, move the muscles away from the spine from the trapezius to the sacrum – repeat on the other side. This should be a rhythmical rocking motion, using your body weight to lean in and move the muscles.

Spinal Circles

With your thumbs, work down the spine in a circular motion away from the spine from T1 to the base of the sacrum. These circles may be right against the vertebrae and considerable time may be taken over this technique. Use any time in the sequence, but it is particularly useful before working on the nine points with elbow pressure. This can also be speeded up and used to warm up the lower back area.

Lower Back Stretch

All stretches need to be held for a minimum of eight seconds. Place the heel of your left hand (fingers pointing diagonally downwards) on the right iliac crest of the client and your right hand (fingers pointing upwards) on the left scapula. Get the client to take a deep breath, and when they breathe out, stretch on the diagonal with your arms crossed. Repeat this on the opposite side.

The lower back stretch can be adapted to stretch the whole left side of the back, by using the same technique as the diagonal stretch. Keep arms crossed, but have both hands on the same side of the clients' body. Make sure the muscles are warm before you attempt a stretch.

Chronic Neck Tension

Gently tip the head forward and with your fingertips resting on the client's shoulders, work your thumbs up on either side of the cervical spine, from C7 to the occipital base. Be aware of areas of tension and any irregularities in the musculature. If there are, repeat this process whilst slowly moving your thumbs in a circular motion to release any adhesions. You may take your time over this movement.

Continue down the neck and onto the trapezius, circling out towards the shoulder joint, and moving the muscle away from the spine. This will help to remove adhesions around C7 where many people experience stiffness.

Neck Squeeze

Interlace your fingers and turn your palms towards the back of the neck, with your little fingers up against the base of the skull - gently squeeze inwards in three movements, working down the muscles on either side of the cervical vertebrae.

Work along either side of the cervical vertebrae with ascending alternate hand movement, taking the muscle between thumb and forefinger.

Pectoral Circles

Start from just below the clavicle (kidney meridian) and working outwards with your fingertips to the space between the pectorals and deltoid (lung meridian). Massage your fingertips in circular motion all around the anterior rotator cuff muscles.

Chinese Roll

This technique is used extensively in Chinese massage and can be applied to any muscle group anywhere on the body with great effect. Keep the lateral side of the hand in constant contact with the client's muscle. Roll the hand back and forth across the muscle, remaining for several moments on any areas of tension and tightness or at trigger points and acupressure points. This technique is particularly good for working the area where the shoulder and neck meet and also around the rotator cuff muscles.

SOFT TISSUE TRIGGER POINT AND POSITIONAL RELEASE TECHNIQUES

There are well-documented connections between myofascial trigger point activity and a wide range of whole body dysfunctions. Trigger points appear in muscles stressed from postural imbalances and other traumas both physical and psychological. There are several classic positions for trigger point activity in the muscles of the shoulders and neck and they are commonly found in fibrotic tissue, feeling like a hard pea-sized lump under the fingers. The trigger point itself will be painful when palpated, but will also have a target area to which pain or other symptoms are referred. There are several methods of releasing trigger points, but it is important to bring the muscle back to its normal resting length or else the trigger point will come back. Always warm the muscles first before attempting trigger point release. Apply pressure directly onto the trigger point by direct downward pressure with the thumb or compress the trigger point between thumb and forefinger. In many cases moving an associated joint to a position where the muscle is at ease and the discomfort is reduced (positional release) will enhance the effect of trigger point release. When the discomfort disappears, usually after 15-30 seconds, the muscle should be stretched passively to its new length. Another method is for the client to introduce an isometric contraction to the muscle while the trigger point is compressed by the therapist for at least 15 secs.

Sacrum Paddle

In addition to the lower back point work and stretches learned in part 1&2, you can release the lower back further, by standing directly behind the client, tucking your elbows into your waist and using the heels of both hands gently paddle the sacrum and along the iliac crest with downward pushes using alternate hands.

STRETCHING

These exercises can either be done as a complete series, or individually, depending on individual requirements. Some will ease tension in specific parts of the body, whilst others will help with general relaxation. Stretching should be relaxing and never be painful.

The busier you are, the more important it is to make time for relaxation and stretching exercises. A number of these exercises can be carried out at work, during breaks and even at your desk! To get the maximum benefit from these exercises, they must be carried out regularly – preferably each day.

Each stretch must be held for at least 15 to 45 seconds and repeated twice on each side.

Head and Neck
- Head rotation – keeping your head level, slowly turn it from side to side.
- Slowly drop your head sideways moving your right ear towards your right shoulder and push down with your left shoulder. Repeat on the other side.

- Stand with feet shoulder distance apart; look down towards right foot (hold for 15 seconds) dropping left shoulder. Repeat exercise looking towards left foot.
- Drop the lower jaw and open the mouth wide.
- Neck release – This technique can be taught to all your clients who experience stiffness when moving the neck through its range of motion. Ask the client to bend the neck to one side as far as they can go without discomfort. Ask them to tap firmly along the length of the extended sternoclaidomastoid muscle with the tips of their fingers. Repeat on the other side of the neck. With head bent forward and back of neck muscles extended, ask them to tap the muscles on either side of the spine from the top of the shoulders, up the neck and halfway up the back of the head. This stimulates the underused muscle fibres to prepare for action.
- Looking straight ahead, 'draw' small circles in **both directions** with the nose. Turn the head to the left and draw small circles with the chin in **both directions**, repeat on the other side. This isolates and releases the specific muscles that turn and bend the neck. If practised daily, the neck should remain free from stiffness and discomfort.

Shoulders
- Shrugging shoulders in a circular movement – forwards then backwards.
- Raise your shoulders high and let them drop heavily, whilst letting your breath go.
- Clasp hands behind head, with elbows back – push your chin back. Hold. From this position look down and push your elbows together at the front.
- Clasp hands and push up towards ceiling, palms up – look down
- Sit upright in a chair with a firm seat. Raise your arms as high as possible and remaining seated, drop forward letting your head and arms hang heavily towards the floor.

Arms and Hands
- Stand with your feet together, keeping your knees soft. Raise your arms alternately swinging them over your head as if you were performing backstroke.
- Raise your left arm above your head and push up as high as you can. Feel the stretch down the left side of the body. Hold for 30 seconds. Repeat on right.
- Raise your right arm to the side, keeping at shoulder height. Point your

fingers behind you and push your palm away from your body. Hold for 30 seconds and repeat on left side.

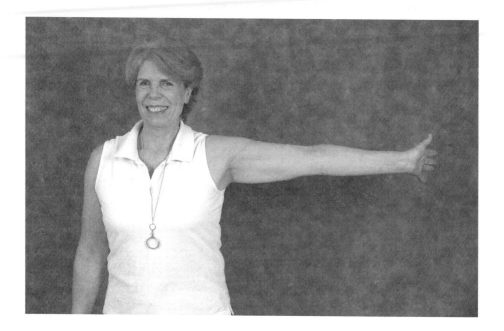

- If you would like to increase the stretch, reach over with your right arm, placing your hand flat around the ear, and gently pull across as shown.

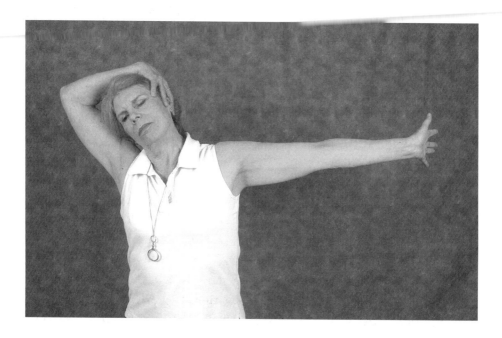

- With your right hand by your side, point your fingers behind you with your palm facing up. Push your right shoulder and wrist towards the floor, then make a fist. Hold. Repeat on the other side.
- Keep your arms by your side and clench your fists as tight as you can, then spread your thumb and fingers as far apart as possible.
- Let your arms hang loosely by your side and shake them for about 15 seconds.

Back

- Clasp elbows in front of your body at shoulder height, making big circle in front of you – push out and look down. This will stretch your upper back.
- Lie on your back and raise your legs with knees bent and hands palms down at right angles to your body. Move your legs over to one side of your body keeping your knees together and bent. Repeat for the other side.

Lumbar stretch

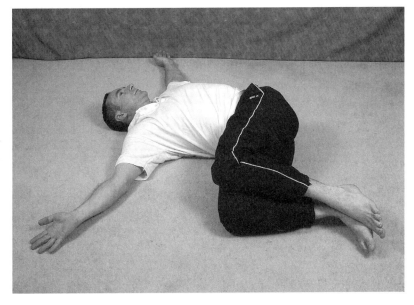

- Lie on your back with arms at right angles to your body. Raise a leg with your knee bent and let it drop over to the opposite side of your body.
- Sit back with your buttocks on your heels and head on the floor, hands outstretched in front of you. This will stretch the entire length of the spine.
- Kneel on all fours, look down whilst arching your back upwards, then slowly drop your back down and stretch your head up.
- Lie on your back with your right knee up keeping your foot on the ground. Place your left ankle on your right knee, letting your left knee drop outwards. Clasp your hands below your right knee and pull

towards your body. Repeat for the other side. This will stretch the gluteals.

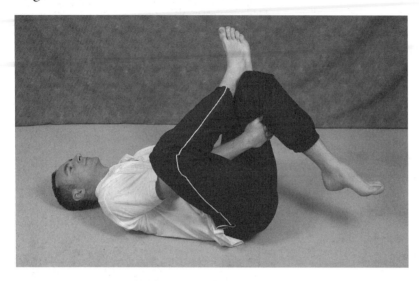

Gluteal stretch

- Lie on your stomach with your arms by your side and gently raise your head slightly, if this feels comfortable then you can also raise your feet off the ground and raise your arms above your head in front of you. This is especially useful for straight backs and good for strengthening.
- Sit with your right leg straight in front of you. Drop your left knee to the floor as you bend your left leg, bringing your left heel as high up your right thigh as possible. Sit as upright as you can and raise your left arm, lean forward from the hips as you rotate your upper body to the right, bringing your left arm to the outside of your right leg. The greater the rotation, the better the stretch. This is known as the 'ballet stretch'.

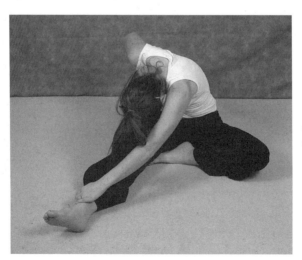

Ballet stretch

- Sit with your legs straight in front of you. Bend your right knee and place your right foot on the floor to the outside of your left knee. Rotate your upper body to the right, and place your left elbow (arm straight) on the outside of your right knee, with your right hand supporting yourself behind your back. This will stretch your gluteals and lower back.

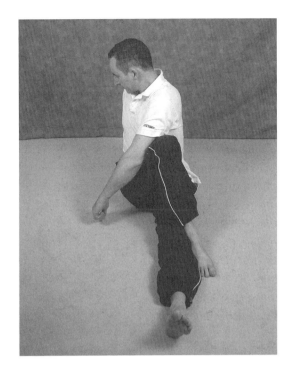

LEGS

Quadriceps

Bend your knee behind you and holding your ankle. Support yourself to keep your balance and keep your knees together and move your hips forward until you feel a stretch. Repeat each side twice.

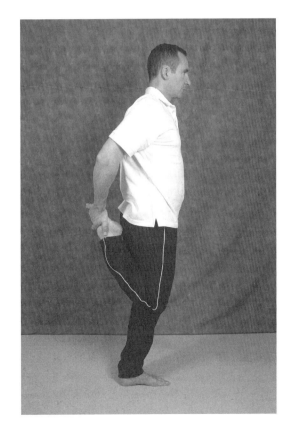

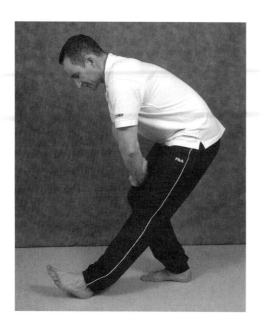

Hamstrings

If it is not appropriate to lie on the floor, this hamstring stretch is simple to perform. To stretch the right hamstring, place most of your weight on your left leg and bend your knee. Bring your right leg in front of you and keep it straight. Bend at the waist slightly and rest your hands on your left knee, sink down further to increase the stretch.

DO-IN

A self-massage routine to stimulate all the major meridians

This is a great routine for us as massage practitioners before we start work, but it is also a suitable one to show your clients for their self-help programme. It only takes a few minutes to do, it's fun and the seriously busy people who work long hours might be willing to squeeze the sequence into their crowded daily schedule.

Stand with your feet hip-width apart and take a few deep breaths. Make a loose fist with your right hand and starting on the left shoulder, rhythmically 'punch' the muscles around the body as follows:

- Down the outside of left arm to hand.
- Turn hand palm upwards and continue back up inside of arm to armpit (these are Ying channels so 'punch' slightly more gently).
- Down the left side of body and continue down outside of left leg, across the top of the foot and back up inside of leg to the groin.
- Down the inside of the right leg over the foot and up the outside of the right leg
- Continue up the right side of the body and down the inside of the right arm to the hand.

- Turn the right hand palm up and continue up the outside of the right arm across the top of the right shoulder.
- Beat the chest with loose fists.
- Beat the head – gently – with loose fists, starting at the top of the head at the hairline and working across the top and down to the base of the skull
- Bend over and using the back of your fist work down either side of the spine to the gluteal muscles.
- Starting at your hands, shake your hands and arms loosely.
- Lift one leg at a time and shake loosely.
- Take three deep breaths and brush down the front and back of your body with open palms.

You will feel your energy surging round your body, you will be relaxed and clear-headed and ready to deal with your day.

DO-IN FLOW

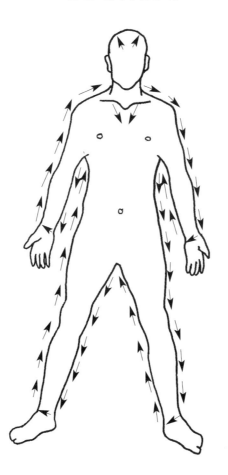

AFTERCARE ADVICE FOR CLIENTS

Acupressure therapy is a non-invasive treatment, which can help reduce the effects of stress and promote a sense of well-being. Regular treatments have a cumulative effect and provide greater benefit than an individual session.

After the treatment, you should feel relaxed but energised and alert. You may experience some mild, short-lived reactions as your body responds to the therapy. You may feel light-heated, your muscles may ache, you might feel hot or cold and you might have an emotional release.

In order to assist your body to eliminate toxins after your treatment, please follow this general advice:

- Relax as much as possible
- Drink plenty of plain water
- Eat a light diet
- Reduce tea, coffee and alcohol

Your practitioner will discuss with you other long-term adjustments you could make to manage stress by simple health promoting measures.

A FINAL WORD

Last but not least – A few reminders about your health and well-being as a practitioner.

- Pace yourself! Don't get carried away with the excitement of securing your first company contract and overextend yourself. Build in breaks for yourself between treatments and try not to work on more than ten 30-minute appointments per day or you will 'burn out'. Two or three days per week at that pace is enough for any practitioner of seated acupressure therapy.
- For peace of mind, have a reliable colleague to back you up if you need a day off.
- Always eat breakfast.
- Drink plenty of water.
- Eat a well balanced diet, with plenty of 'slow-burning foods' when you are working.
- Always stretch and ground yourself before starting treatments.
- Get a regular treatment for yourself.
- You are promoting health, be a good rôle model for your clients and look after yourself.

Chapter 7
Marketing Yourself As A Practitioner

MANAGING YOUR BUSINESS

Traditionally, practitioners are reluctant to see themselves as business people, and in the early days of building a practice, many of us even feel uncomfortable about asking for our fee at the end of a treatment. That improves with time of course, but practitioners of seated acupressure therapy who are planning to secure contracts in the business world, do not have time to be coy about the value of the service they are offering. When approaching a company with your proposal, you need to be professional and confident.

Preparation is the key to success in any business and that means sitting down and writing a business plan and setting up a simple book-keeping system. If you need help with this, in the UK, many banks and organisations have excellent, 'Starting or Running Your Business' packs, or you can contact your local Enterprise Council and local Business Link for help. Look into attending courses on starting and running a business. Work out the costs of training, therapy chair and advertising costs. The local Inland Revenue Office will give you guidance on your tax returns and National Insurance payments.

If you want to borrow money from the bank to set up your business, you need to present a business plan to them, but even if you are not borrowing money, a business plan will help you to stay focused about your own goals. Before you start to write your business plan, it might help you to think about the following points.

Business Name
Does it give you the right image? Avoid using the word massage in your business name.

Business/Personal History
What experience do you have for this activity?

Personal Aims and Objectives
What do you want from the business apart from profit?

Aims and Objectives of the Business
Where do you want it to be in a few years time?

In addition, think about key people, market research, advertising and promotion plans, premises and equipment, on-going training, relevant legal matters such as contracts or consumer laws and financial structure, capital, survival income and first three years profit projection. In short, your plan should include:

- Statement of overall business aims. Keep it short and specific.
- Target market e.g. private or business sector.
- Why your product/service is special.
- Resources that you will need.
- What price you will charge and how have you determined it.
- How you will promote your business.
- Set-up costs, fixed monthly costs, cash flow.
- General book-keeping.

You cannot manage your money if you do not know how much you are earning or where it is going, so keeping accurate and up-to-date records and accounts is important. You are required to keep them by law, but they are vital for calculating your tax returns. There is no need for a complicated system, just use common sense. The basics include:

1. A concertina-type file – divide the sections into months and keep all your business-related receipts in the relevant month's partition.
2. An accounts ledger – record all your purchase items for the tax year,

month by month in one section. Number your receipts and record the number against the purchase item. Show your income month by month in another section and make up your own record of expenses and income and keep it updated. Reconcile purchases and payments with your monthly bank statement.

3. You may not be VAT registered to begin with but keep a VAT column going. If your business grows to a point where you have to register, then you can claim VAT for two retrospective years.

GROWING YOUR BUSINESS

This may be on a purely local basis, or on a national scale for the more ambitious therapist wanting to set up an agency network. Here are some ideas:

A computer

A computer is now essential in running your own business from home – whether it is for letters, invoicing or making power point presentations. Keeping in touch with clients by email is the easiest mode of communication in business – if you have not already set yourself up with an email address, now is the time. There are many courses offered by local Colleges, which will de-mystify emails and the internet. Professional flyers and leaflets can be produced inexpensively and effectively on your own system.

A Website

Having your own web site does not need to cost and arm and a leg. It is your own on-line brochure, and one that will never go out of date and have to be thrown away because of changes in information. Many web sites give you the facility to be able to edit and update the information yourself. Of course the more sophisticated the site, the more it will cost, but any web site address can be printed on your business cards for clients to read about your therapies and services.

Talks and Presentations

Perfect your presentation skills, and reach a large number of potential clients and referral services, by offering free talks or demonstrations. This may either be prepared as a power point presentation, or printed in colour and placed in a folder, in sequence, to guide you through your presentation. Remember to plan your talk, involve or engage the audience and keep it clear and interesting. Some places you may target could be:

- G.P's surgeries
- Women's Institute
- Sports clubs
- Residential care homes, hospices and hospitals
- Social clubs
- Lunch-hour presentations in companies for staff

Exhibitions

You may wish to spend a proportion of your marketing budget on an exhibition. First make sure that it really is the target market you wish to attract. Then, having spent money on the stand space, it is essential that your stand is interesting and professional.

- Produce literature, and have it blown up to poster size and mounted on art board, or laminated.
- Have special exhibition offer discounts on treatments, as this will generate a great deal of interest and you will soon have a queue of people waiting to try the therapy.
- Have back-up and fellow practitioners that can help you on the day – it is important to acknowledge each person that shows and interest in your stand, and this may be difficult to do if you are working on a client.
- Have cards and information to hand out and make sure you take the details of each person who could be a potential client.

HELPFUL TIPS TO PROMOTE YOURSELF WITHIN THE CORPORATE SECTOR

Target Market

Identify the types of company you are going to contact and formulate a package tailored to their requirements. It may be an area in which you have a particular interest, or an environment where you have previously worked, so that you can personalise it. It is much easier to 'sell' something that you have a better knowledge of.

Collecting Information

Find out as much as you can about the company that you are going to see – either before you visit, or when you begin the meeting. Don't just try to sell your service before finding out what problems the staff and employers are having. What levels of stress are the staff under? Does the company have shift workers? How many employees do they have? What other services do they offer to their employees to reduce stress? What sort of hours do the staff work at the VDU's? Do they have a problem with absenteeism, RSI, back pain, etc?

Look Professional

Have brochures and business cards printed. Make up a folder with some information to support your presentation. It is a good idea to leave some information on what you do and a scale of fees. It is also beneficial if you can work with someone else, even if it is only someone who covers for you if you are on holiday or sick, as organisations are sometimes reluctant to deal with just one individual.

Pricing

When you present your costs, be confident. Remember the service you are offering may end up *saving the company money*. Make sure you have thought out pricing carefully, so that you know what the cost per head is. If the company asks you for something you have not calculated, or you feel like you have been put on the spot and are not good with figures, write down what they require, and tell them you will send them a written quotation when you have calculated it.

HANDLING OBJECTIONS

We Have Group Medical Health Insurance

Medical health insurance is a necessity when it comes to giving people peace of mind and immediate medical attention if required – however it does not offer practical stress management and is rather like 'closing the stable door, after the horse has bolted'.

We Offer Telephone Counselling Services/Individual Counselling

Many people are unaware of their stress levels, so would not consider confronting issues with counsellors, whilst others may feel that it is admitting weakness to do so.

We Have Company Gym Membership

It is known that although this is a valuable service for those that use it, only 10% of individuals within a company take advantage of these services. Not surprisingly, the employees who use the gym are generally those that least need help.

We Offer Stress Management Seminars

Like any seminars or sales training, these are usually very informative and enable people to understand what happens to the body during a stressful event and they are given tools to deal with it. The seminars may also 'kick-start' an individual to make some life changes, some of which may be extremely helpful. Unfortunately, like New Year resolutions, they are often forgotten. The seminars cannot really replace the sort of regular one-on-one attention a practitioner would be able to provide within the workplace.

We Have Company Doctors

Although the employee is assured of first-class medical attention, many problems could be prevented or otherwise dealt with immediately, thus eliminating the need for a visit, additional expense and time out of the office.

The subject of stress in the workplace has been discussed elsewhere in this book. This information will help practitioners formulate a concise, corporate presentation.

In the ordinary private lives of employees within a company, one may be sure that there are already a number who are experiencing high levels of stress. For example those who are divorced, single parents, or unhappily married. Those contending with bereavement, chronic illness, changes in line of work, additional workload or fear of redundancy. Additional stress will place those people in a high-risk category. Judgments about who is the most likely to be unable to cope with added stress are not easy to make – even for the individual themselves.

Stress is known to be a contributor in ninety per cent of disease and illness. A good stress reduction programme can mean fewer lost days at work. Some of the less well-known aspects of stress are the mental and emotional components. These range from forgetfulness, feeling angry, loss of confidence, lack of concentration, problems in making decisions, irritability, depression, withdrawal, feeling explosive, guilt, hopelessness, panic attacks and anxiety, to list only a few. Seated Acupressure Therapy can help alleviate the symptoms of:

- Anxiety and depression.
- Eyestrain.
- Sinus problems.
- Headaches and migraines.
- Insomnia.
- Backache and sciatica (both recent and old injuries).
- Muscular tension.
- Asthma and breathing difficulties.
- Chronic Fatigue Syndrome.
- Repetitive Strain Injury and Carpal Tunnel Syndrome (including the onset or mild symptoms such as tingling, pins and needles and numbness in hands and fingers).
- Menstrual tension.
- Neck tension and whiplash injuries.
- Skin problems (psoriasis, eczema).
- Hypertension.
- Irritable Bowel Syndrome and digestive problems.

It is not unknown for employees suffering high levels of stress or RSI, to sue their employers. To protect the company from the possibility of litigation, the employer must be seen to be addressing this issue. Effective stress management means having a range of ways to reduce stress. In-house treatment would complement the services companies may already offer to staff.

For part of your presentation, you could summarise the corporate benefits on introducing seated acupressure massage as follows:

- Reduces absenteeism.
- Improves morale.
- Demonstrates commitment of management to staff.
- Practical stress management with immediate results.
- Increases productivity.
- SAVES money.

Glossary of Terms

Anma   The art of Japanese massage.

Circadian Rhythm   24-hour biological clock.

Cosmological Sequence   Sequence of the five elements in the body.

CTD   Cumulative Trauma Disorders.

CTS   Carpal Tunnel Syndrome.

CVS   Computer Vision Syndrome.

De Quervain's   A type of Carpal Tunnel Syndrome.
Tenovaginitis

Ergonomics   An applied science concerned with
                                  designing and arrangement of work
                                  environments to create maximum safety,
                                  comfort and efficiency for the worker.

Fight or Flight Mechanism   The body's release of hormones such as
                                  adrenaline and noradrenalin in response
                                  to a stressful challenge.

Five Element Theory   Taoist philosophy relating health to
                                  Growth and Control cycles of Earth,
                                  Wood, Fire, Water and Metal.

Holmes-Rahe Stress Scale   Graded scale of stressful events in life.

Huang Ti Ne Ching	Oldest existing medical text in the world.
Kata	Dance or form, used to describe the formalized moves of the 20-minute seated acupressure massage sequence. Also used in marshal arts and Tai Chi.
Ke Cycle Theory	Control Cycle of the Five Element.
Meridians	Interconnecting pathways carrying Qi (energy) to all parts of the body.
Qi or Ki (pronounced chee)	Universal life force or energy flowing through the meridians.
RSI	Repetitive Strain Injury.
Shen	Spirit.
Sheng Cycle Theory	Growth Cycle of the Five Element.
Shiatsu	'Finger pressure' massage, a derivative of Anma, now a separate discipline.
TCM	Traditional Chinese Medicine.
Tsubo	Means vase or jar in Chinese and describes the acupressure points found near the surface on the major meridians.
Types of Qi	Congenital Qi, essence of life inherited from parents at birth. Acquired Qi, derived from food we eat and air we breathe. These two combine to create Meridian Qi, Defensive Qi and Nourishing Qi. Qi in turn supports the circulation and formation of blood.

Ultradian Rhythm   The body's need for movement and a change of activity every 90 minutes.

WRULD   Work-related upper limb disorders.

Yin and Yang   Opposite and balancing aspects of all of life e.g. night and day, male and female, cold and hot etc.

Recommended Further Reading

Jarmey, Chris and Tindall, John: *Acupressure for Common Ailments,* Gaia Books 1991, ISBN 1-85675-015-9.

Mercati, Maria: *Step-by-Step Tuina,* Gaia Books Ltd 1997, ISBN 1-85675-038-8.

Pyves, G: "No Hands Massage –Zero-Strain Bodywork" and **Pyves, G, Woodhouse, D**: *No Hands Chair Massage,* Shi'Zen Publications 2000, ISBN 0-9539074-0-6 and 0-9539074-1-4.

Rich, G.J: *Massage Therapy, The evidence for practice,* Mosby 2002, ISBN 0-7234-3217-1.

Hix, S. and Batten, J: *Fourteen Classical Meridian Charts,* Roswell Publications 1998, ISBN 0-953-3850-0-0.

Connelly, D: *Traditional Acupuncture, The Law of the Five Elements,* Traditional Acupuncture Institute 1994, ISBM 0-912381-0305.

Bibliography and References

Mochizuki, Shogo: *Anma the Art of Japanese Massage*,
Kotobuki Publications, 1999.

Williams, Tom: *Chinese Medicine*, Time Life Books, 1996.

Chalmers Mill, Wendy: *Chartered Physiotherapist Repetitive Strain Injury*,
Thorsons Health Series (out of print).

Repetitive Strain Injury Association: *Newsletters*,
RSI Association, 1998-2005.

Silk, Anne: *Air Quality and the Workplace of the Future*, Mid Career
College Press, 1999.

Confederation of British Industry: *CBI Focus on Absence Survey
Health and Safety Commission*, Health and Safety Statistics
Government Statistical Service, 1998.

Health and Safety Executive: *Good Health is Good Business*,
HSE, 1995.

Lewith, George T: *Acupuncture – Its Place in Western Medical Science*,
Thorsons Publishing Group.

American Optometric Association: *The Effects of Video Display Terminal Use on Eye Health and Vision*, AOA, Revised 1997.

Harvey E and Oatley, M.J: *Acupressure*, Headway

McDonald, E: *Work and Disease*, Update 1996.

Gill, C.R.W: *Repetitive Strain Injury*, Update 1996.

Useful Addresses

Seated Acupressure Therapy Training School
82 The Spinney
Beaconsfield
Bucks HP9 1SA
Tel 01494 764666 or 678221
Fax: 01494 681284
Email info@acupressure-training.co.uk
www.acupressure-training.co.uk

The Academy of Seated Acupressure (On-Site) Massage
New St
Charfield
Wotton-under-Edge
Gloucestershire
GL12 8ES
Tel/Fax 01453 521530

Embody
PO Box 6955
Towcester
NN12 6WZ
info@embody.uk.net

City and Guilds
1 Guiltspur St
London
EC1A 9DD
www.city-and-guilds.co.uk

Confederation of British Industry
http://www.cbi.org.uk

Repetitive Strain Industry Association
The Repetitive Strain Industry Association does not exist any longer but all their information and research can be accessed from the website hosting service: http://rsi.webhosting-services.co.uk/index.asp

Health and Safety Executive
The Health and Safety Executive is also a resource for the latest statistics on stress-related workplace absenteeism. Visit their website: http://www.hse.gov.uk

FURTHER SOURCES OF INFORMATION

There are several models of acupressure therapy chairs available. Approach a training school first as most will offer a student discount.

For a list of companies/agencies offering employment to practitioners of seated acupressure therapy, please contact the **Seated Acupressure Therapy Training School** for details.

Appendix

Client Record Form
(please print clearly)

Name: _____

Address: _____

_____

Email: _____ Tel: _____

DOB: _____

GP/Practice: _____

Tel: _____

To ensure suitability to receive treatment, please answer the following questions:

This sequence is not suitable for anyone who is pregnant or likely to be.

Current Medical Treatment: Details: _____

_____

Blood Pressure: High/Low/Medication: Details: _____

Other medication	YES	NO
Spinal injuries/degenerative diseases	YES	NO
Physical injuries or recent operations	YES	NO
Diabetes	YES	NO
Circulatory problems (i.e. varicose veins/thrombosis)	YES	NO
History of epilepsy	YES	NO
Any on-going medical condition	YES	NO
Digestive/IBS	YES	NO
Allergies	YES	NO

Breathing difficulties	YES	NO

Skin disorders	YES	NO

Is there anything else we should know?   YES   NO
(i.e. any condition that is not covered above)
Please give details: _____
_____
_____

Are you seeing another practitioner for anything at present?   YES   NO

Practitioner, please check each time if client has eaten.

What would you like to achieve from these treatments? Please give details: _____
_____
_____
_____

LIFESTYLE

Smoking: YES   NO   Alcohol: YES   NO
If yes, quantity: _____   Units per week: _____

Any special diet? _____

Exercise: _____

Stress Levels: _____

Occupation: _____

I understand the nature of the treatment as explained to me by the Practitioner. I have answered the above questions to the best of my knowledge and will inform the Practitioner when attending further treatments if there is any change to my medical history. I am aware that this treatment is not a substitute for medical advice.

_____   _____
Signature   Print Name

Practitioner's Name: _____

Treatment Record
(These details will remain Private and Confidential)

Client Ref: _____

Treatment Date: _____

Response to previous treatment: _____
_____
_____
_____
_____
_____

Practitioner findings: _____
_____
_____
_____
_____
_____

Treatment given: _____
_____
_____
_____
_____
_____

Response to this treatment: _____
_____
_____

Recommendations: _____

Additional Notes: _____

Index

Notes

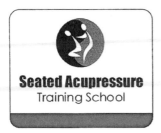 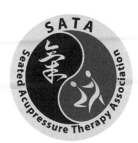

About The School

The Seated Acupressure Therapy Training School courses are accredited by City and Guilds at Level 3 and approved by EMBODY and the Association of Complementary Therapists. We are also founder members of SATA (Seated Acupressure Therapy Association), part of Seated Acupressure professionals who set the standards for all EMBODY-approved Seated Acupressure Therapy courses. Graduates of the School receive a Certificate in Seated Acupressure Therapy from City and Guilds and a Diploma from the School. Insuranace cover is offered by EMBODY and other leading professional therapists' organizations.

Courses are offered throughout the year in the UK and details about courses, training videos or CDs can be obtained by contacting the school:
Website: www.acupressure-training.co.uk
Email: info@acupressure-training.co.uk
Telephone: 01494 764666/678221
Fax: 01494 681284
Write to: The Seated Acupressure Therapy Training School
82, The Spinney,
Beaconsfield,
Bucks,
HP9 1SA.

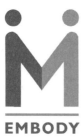

EMBODY

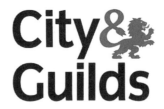